Ageing

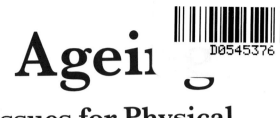

Issues for Physical, Psychological and Social Health

Edited by

PHILIP WOODROW

Practice Development Nurse, Kent & Canterbury Hospital

W

WHURR PUBLISHERS
LONDON AND PHILADELPHIA

First published 2002 by
Whurr Publishers Ltd
19b Compton Terrace, London N1 2UN, England and
325 Chestnut Street, Philadelphia PA 19106, USA

Reprinted 2005

British Library Cataloguing in Publication Data
A catalogue record for this book is available from the British
Library.

ISBN: 1 86156 311 6

Printed and bound in the UK by Athenaeum Press Ltd,
Gateshead, Tyne & Wear

Contents

About the authors

Stephen Cook, Senior Lecturer at the School of Health, Biological and Environmental Sciences (HeBES), Middlesex University.

Dympna Crowley, Senior Lecturer at the School of Health, Biological and Environmental Sciences (HeBES), Middlesex University.

Kate Davidson, the Centre for Research on Ageing and Gender (CRAG), the Department of Sociology, University of Surrey.

Nicky Hayes, Consultant Nurse in the Healthcare of Older People Department, King's College Hospital, Dulwich.

Henry Minardi, Senior Lecturer at the School of Health, Biological and Environmental Sciences (HeBES), Middlesex University.

Mary Tilki, Principal Lecturer, School of Health, Biological and Environmental Sciences (HeBES), Middlesex University.

Philip Woodrow, Practice Development Nurse (Critical Care), East Kent Hospital, NHS Trust.

Preface

Much has been written about healthcare for older people, but the ageing process affects people of all ages. Ageing, rather than old people, has received limited attention within healthcare literature. This book is primarily about ageing, although inevitably age-related issues usually become more significant for older people, and those involved with their healthcare, than for younger generations.

This book is written for people studying and working in a range of healthcare professions. This diversity is reflected in the range of authors contributing to this text. Healthcare relies on teamwork between a range of professionals. Increased range and complexity of needs among older people make multi-professional teamwork especially important for the healthcare of older people.

In a text such as this, deciding whether to use more technical or more familiar terms can be problematic. Because health professionals will need a reasonable understanding of technical terminology for their own practice, many technical terms are included in this text. However, where these are obscure, they have been clarified either in the text or in the glossary at the end of the book.

The health needs and problems of older people can be complex. Some topics and issues are inevitably covered in more than one chapter. For example, falls, which are a major cause of hospitalization and death among older people, may be the result of a wide range of problems. Cross-references are included to help readers find any relevant material in other chapters.

Any book is a team effort, and I am grateful to everyone in the team that has brought this book into existence. I have been fortunate in being able to gather a team of authors who have a breadth of expertise and experience. I would also like to thank Tim Bettsworth, both for picking up my typographical errors and helping develop and clarify the text. I am especially grateful to Jim McCarthy, who first suggested the idea of this book and without whose support this book would not have been written, and to the rest of the team at Whurr.

Philip Woodrow
January 2002

CHAPTER 1

What is ageing?

PHILIP WOODROW

This book explores key perspectives on the ageing process. 'Ageing' and 'old' are not necessarily interchangeable terms; meanings may vary according to the context in which they are used.

Ageing is something that affects us all, whether or not we are 'old'. Ageing is a process that begins the day we are born and only ends when we die. The effects of ageing have obsessed most people for at least as long as records exist. When people think about ageing, it is often viewed negatively, as something to be halted and, if possible, reversed. Considerable time and money have been spent searching for an 'elixir of youth'. Yet any elixir remains elusive.

In contrast, 'old' is a relative term, applied (explicitly or implicitly) when comparing an 'older' with a 'younger' person. So, for example, 'older' may be applied to children when comparing different age groups among them (e.g. at school).

The focus of most discussion in this book is 'ageing' rather than 'old', but, as most readers are likely to be caring for 'older' people, special application is made to the older cohorts among our society.

Why is ageing important?

The population of the UK and most countries in the world is growing older. As the number of old people increases, the demands on healthcare systems will increase. Care of older people, however defined, is not just an issue for staff working on designated wards for older people. Most older people in hospital are not in departments designated specifically for 'old' people (Tinker 1997, Masterson 1999). So nearly all health professionals, apart from those on children's wards, care for older people. Healthcare for older people has long been grossly under-valued. As the number of older people increases, knowledge of ageing, its effects and implications, will become increasingly necessary for most healthcare staff.

However, this book is not simply about older people. The ageing process is something that is constantly affecting every person. While normal ageing is inevitable, abnormal ageing and disease processes are not. Many people fear that an increased life expectancy means longer years of severe disability in old age (Simons et al 2000). Although these fears are often unfounded, they are understandable. Ageing is something that can affect, or be feared by, people of any age.

Visible signs of body changes (e.g. puberty, menopause) can appear threatening. For older people, baldness or greying/whitening of hair form similarly visible rites of passage, with the added disadvantage of usually being obvious to everyone they meet. Changes in appearance may be relatively insignificant as far as biological health is concerned but can significantly affect a person's self-concept, or the way they are treated by others. Therefore, ageing (and its effects) should be considered when caring (and planning care) for any person.

De Beauvoir (1970) suggests that three distinct approaches to the study of ageing have developed:

- physiological
- chronological
- sociological.

Physiology defines age by the person's (biological) ability to function. Chronology defines age by the number of years lived. Sociology defines age by one's role in society. This classification provides a useful means to explore perspectives on ageing; so each theme is introduced in this chapter. Chronological ageing is discussed below but is not developed as a theme within this book.

Physiological ageing

Throughout adulthood there is a progressive decline of all physiological functions, although the rate of decline varies between functions and between individuals. Physiological decline can make for depressing study and can encourage stereotyping of older people as being malfunctional or disease-ridden. Both of these problems can be avoided by remembering that most older people are healthy.

Considering the vast number of cells that make up the human body, surprisingly few problems will occur within the human lifetime. But problems can and do occur, causing ill health, some of which may be preventable. For much of most people's lives declining function will usually be insignificant and unnoticeable, but, as we become older, that process accelerates. The interaction of body systems means that the decline of one system can affect others.

In health, each system normally has, at birth, a significant *reserve function*. Reserve function is the ability of a system to function beyond the minimum level needed to maintain homeostasis. For example, at birth most people's pancreatic function can meet any demands placed on it. But pancreatic function progressively declines throughout life. In later life some people will no longer produce sufficient insulin to meet the needs created by an unregulated diet. This lack of sufficient insulin that can occur in later life is called type 2 (or sometimes 'late-onset') diabetes mellitus. Reducing the sugar and starch intake from diets may be sufficient to restore homeostasis, although some people with type 2 diabetes will need oral hypoglycaemic drugs, and a few will need insulin.

Biologically, the body seeks to maintain homeostasis. Demand placed on tissues varies, but when reserve capacity is small failure becomes more likely. For example, ill health places additional stress on most body systems. Illness may be enough to cause system failure. With recovery, demand on that system is usually reduced; so it may regain its pre-illness level of reserve function. For example, someone with chronic respiratory disease may have sufficient function to cope with normal daily activities, albeit with limited function. But a chest infection will further reduce their respiratory function and may cause respiratory failure, which may result in hospitalization.

While this book describes potential physiological decline, it is important to remember that most body systems in most people will maintain an adequate reserve function to support their needs. As long as systems can meet the person's needs, the person may be considered healthy. When the ability of one system fails to meet their minimum needs, they may be considered (physiologically) unhealthy.

Physiological systems within the body have matured by early life, many by birth. However, during life we learn to develop and use our body. This process of adaptation can also occur when some function has been lost (for example following a stroke). Therefore, people who have chronic health problems often consider themselves to be 'well', despite labels of chronic diseases. When asked, these people may not immediately identify problems that they have adapted or adjusted to. Health professionals should therefore make a thorough assessment to identify chronic as well as acute problems.

The section dealing with physiological ageing in this book includes some discussion of normal bodily functions and some pathologies that can result when physiological ageing reduces function. However, this book focuses on applied physiology rather than pure anatomy or medical pathophysiology. Issues raised by these chapters may, therefore, need to be pursued further by readers, according to their individual needs. There are many good anatomy and medical pathophysiology texts, some of which are included in the reference lists, that can meet these needs. Knowledge of biological ageing can help health professionals plan health promotion; many issues discussed in the first section of this book are developed in Chapter 14.

There have been many theories about why the body ages. Theories that are currently more influential are reviewed in Chapter 2, with detailed discussion of Hayflick's 'body clock' theory, subsequent work on apoptosis and free-radical theories of ageing. Explanation of the body clock, apoptosis and free-radical theories necessitates some discussion of normal and abnormal cell function.

Most chapters in this first section describe specific body systems. The ageing of each system affects the function of many other systems. While reductionism provides a useful framework to study and assess ageing, this chapter concludes by emphasizing the importance of holistic care.

Physiological ageing is most easily understood by describing individual body systems. So Chapter 3 describes musculo-skeletal and skin ageing, Chapter 4 shows how the cardiovascular system ages and Chapter 5 gives a brief overview of ageing of other main body systems. These chapters develop some related issues, such as diet and smoking. To end this section of the book, Chapter 6 explores how the senses are affected by ageing.

Chronological ageing

The chronological identification of ageing is widely used in Western societies. Chronological ageing classifies someone as being 'old' because they have reached a certain chronological age (e.g. 65 years). Viewed chronologically, old age occurs when (and if) people approach the upper end of their life expectancy. So old age would vary in different historical periods or different societies. In the Middle Ages, life expectancy (for most people) was around 40–50 years. In Western countries today this has nearly doubled, and people aged 50 are seldom considered to be 'old'.

Although life expectancy can be increased by removing or reducing factors that cause early mortality, there seems to be an upper limit for human life of around one hundred and twenty years (Lueckenotte 2000). Most Western countries are close to achieving this upper limit for many people. Therefore, unless life expectancy changes, concepts of chronological old age will probably not be significantly changed in Western societies. However, in poorer countries changes can (and often are) being made to reduce early mortality. Therefore, globally, concepts of chronological older age are changing.

With current upper limits of life reaching up to around one hundred and twenty years, if the age of 65 is taken to define the beginning of old age, 'old people' includes generations born thirty to forty years apart. Older people are therefore often divided into 'young old' (often 65–75), 'middle old' (75–85) and 'old old' (85+). Such categories can hamper the provision of suitable healthcare.

The use of chronological age is popular, especially for statistics. The benefit for research and statistical analysis is obvious: someone either is or is not over 65. However, their value for healthcare is less clear; comparing 'an old 55' to 'a young 75' illustrates how human individuality often conflicts with the rigidity of chronology, although ironically can reinforce the stereotyping it seeks to overcome.

Rationing health care by imposing minimum or maximum age limits is one way that society uses chronological ageing. For example, many wards catering specifically for older people have a minimum age limit. The danger of rationing health by chronological age is that it is almost inevitably ageist. Rationing by age limit may ensure that appropriate amounts or types of services are provided but more often limits funding, quality or access to services for older people. Although the quality of healthcare environments has improved since Wells' (1980) classic study, some wards and hospitals for older people are still converted workhouses rather than purpose-built, and the quality of staff, and therefore of care, attracted to work in some areas catering for older people can still be negatively affected by poor funding, other limitations to resources, and by stigmatization.

Despite widespread use of chronology, age is more usefully measured by the physical, mental and social functioning of individuals (Scrutton 1992). The value of chronology for healthcare being dubious, it is not developed further as a theme in this book. However, chronological ageing is widely used in statistics and research and so is inevitably included in the discussion of other perspectives.

Psychological ageing

Mental health is an important component of holistic health. It can be affected by various sociological factors. It may also be affected by physiological changes within the brain. While stereotypes of dementia are familiar, the extent of mental health problems experienced by older people often goes unrecognized. Problems may be acute or chronic; so, before labelling someone as 'confused', any possible acute causes (such as hypoxia) should be excluded. Discussion of 'normal' and 'abnormal' psychological ageing is developed in the second section of this book.

This second section is divided into two chapters, the first discusses normal psychological ageing while the second explores abnormal psychological ageing. This division necessitates chapters that are slightly longer than those elsewhere in this book.

Chapter 7 outlines the models and theories of normal psychological ageing, with special focus on the influential work of Erikson. The significance of cognitive, social, political and personal factors across the life-span are explored. Possible changes to normal psychological development through age are identified, providing a context for some of the myths about psychological aspects of ageing, with a focus on their implications for healthcare. Understanding these myths enables healthcare staff to provide more effective healthcare by understanding how ageing affects psychological growth, which might challenge their earlier (erroneous) assumptions about ageing.

Chapter 8 provides a context for abnormal psychology and psychopathology through studies of older people within community settings. Ways in which socio-cultural and biological aspects can negatively affect psychological development are discussed, and ways in which perceptions of socio-cultural and biological factors affect care are analysed.

Many aspects included in other sections of this book, particularly sociological ageing, affect psychological health. For example, labelling influences psychological health and healthcare. Similarly, the divisions between general (i.e. physiological) and mental health are often less clear than healthcare provision might suggest. Although hospitals, hospital wards, nursing homes and healthcare qualifications are often designated either to be 'general' or 'mental' health, older people are even more likely than younger people to have needs in both areas. So staff should consider all the needs of the people they work with and care for.

Sociological ageing

If a person acts as an older person is expected (by others) to act, they may, from a sociological perspective, be considered 'old'. There are various markers that may be used to measure sociological ageing. Some of these markers may be imposed by social norms and structures (such as retirement) and others by historical actions or accident. A person's sociological age and status may significantly affect their health (or vice versa), particularly their mental health, but criteria for measuring sociological age can be particularly problematic.

Most Western societies value productivity; so, while people remain productive, they are not usually considered sociologically old. Productivity is acknowledged with reward (money); so, when people become sociologically old with retirement, they become less able to participate in a consumer-orientated society. Sociological age has close links with chronological age (retirement age usually being 60 or 65), although the increasing trend towards early retirement and the employment of 'pensioners' has confused this perspective. Logically, if older age is equated with retirement from work, a pensioner returning to employment would suddenly become 'un-old' – a clear absurdity.

History has influenced patterns of immigration into, and emigration from, the UK. Many immigrants are from countries that were formerly part of the British Empire. Further examples of historical factors are developed in chapter 9, with retirement used to illustrate sociological ageing.

Labelling people as 'old' may provide a useful way to manage information, but labels can manipulate public attitudes. Labels dehumanize the individual, making it easier, and potentially acceptable, for society to deny their moral rights. Labelling people as 'old' also potentially ignores unpaid productivity (such as voluntary work). Paid work obviously affects income and so the kind of lifestyle that can be afforded. But work usually also provides an opportunity to meet other people.

Each person has an individual set of values, attitudes and beliefs. In part, individual values are developed from values shared by our peers and those promoted by people in authority, especially during childhood. Therefore, although each person will have their own individual set of values, there are certain values that tend to be shared among members of a particular generation. The differing values of different generations can cause problems for health professionals providing care for a different generation of people, such as older age groups. While healthcare usually attempts to avoid overt ageism, covert ageism can too often adversely affect the quality of care.

Chapter 9 shows how the growing awareness and study of ageing during the twentieth century led to the development of various sociological theories, including disengagement theory and symbolic interactionism. The language used within a society has a powerful influence on attitudes, with some words gaining negative and pejorative connotations. While the repeated use of a single adjective might become tedious, this book generally uses the term 'older person', for reasons identified in Chapter 9.

Chapter 10 explores ethical issues within ageing. Ethical principles are identified and discussed. Autonomy, or the lack of it, can be a particular problem within healthcare for older people. This chapter includes detailed discussion of this issue, focusing on communication and informed consent. From this, ways to assist older people make decisions, and the importance of understanding their moral orientation, are discussed.

Chapter 11 develops issues surrounding ethnicity and ageing, using a model of transcultural skills development to identity and challenge assumptions of homogeneity. It examines the:

- limitations of concepts of ethnicity based on skin colour
- consequent neglect of white minority elders
- migration, settlement and life history of different communities
- differing impacts of gender, class and geography
- impact of racist and ageist stereotypes on health
- access to services, health and social care
- existing knowledge of physical and mental health in multi-ethnic groups
- concepts of respect, expectations of family and care in older age
- the meaning of cultural competence.

Healthcare services are in danger of being culturally insensitive; so the importance of including and empowering older people from multi-ethnic groups within mainstream healthcare services is emphasized.

Chapter 12 explores the range of stereotypes, prejudices and emotions that can surround ageing and old people. 'Ageism' – prejudice based on the age (usually chronological) of a person or group of people – can influence attitudes towards older people. Although many cultures and societies traditionally valued older people for their life experiences and knowledge, modern Western societies devalue older people. These values influence care provided by both professional and lay carers. Understanding ageing provides a way to understand the values and social forces that have contributed to these negative views (and fears) about being old and the care that society (including healthcare) provides for older people.

Attitudes, both within healthcare and society, affect the way older people are treated, usually negatively. The media, especially television, play a major part in influencing attitudes. However, the popular media, such as television, also tend to reflect existing negative attitudes. This therefore perpetuates many of the problems already identified in previous chapters. Chapter 13 shows how current and recent media presentation of older people has influenced the attitudes of society.

Chapter 14 explores the meaning of 'living well' in relation to enjoying a good 'quality of life' and how successful ageing can be achieved. Healthcare workers (in hospital) can develop prejudiced perspectives on ageing, influenced by contact with so many older people who are ill. But however health is defined, ill older people remain a minority. The *General Household Survey* of 1988 found that most old people consider themselves to be healthy; the 1994 *General Household Survey* found that 39% of over 65s claimed to have good health and a further 38% claimed to have fairly good health (Tinker 1997).

Key factors, including exercise, diet, smoking and other personal lifestyle/environmental issues are related to the principles of health education and health promotion for older people. Opportunities and barriers to successful ageing are considered within the context of broader social, cultural and political factors. The importance of personal autonomy, choice and control are emphasized.

The conclusion reviews key themes from the book, drawing together major implications and recommendations for practice. Differences between ageing and older age are reiterated, and the importance of holistic approaches to care re-emphasized.

Cultural perspectives

This book presents reviews of key themes with ageing by reviewing available literature. However, most of the literature accessible to UK healthcare staff, and so most of the literature referred to in this book, originates from the UK, the USA and, to a lesser extent, from other primarily English-speaking countries. As much of the literature draws on Caucasian perspectives and experiences of healthcare, its cultural sensitivity should be considered when applying it to the care of people from other ethnic origins. Even within Caucasian societies, there is a variety of different cultures, often with different sets of values and beliefs. The value of retaining people's own cultural identity is increasingly being recognized. However, immigration means that various cultures are mixed within a single country.

Healthcare

In creating a text for a range of health professionals, inevitable differences in terminology can create confusion. For example, 'patients', 'clients' and 'people' are sometimes used interchangeably. 'Patients' tends to be used in a hospital context and 'client' in community and mental health services. But ageing is not a disease, and older people are not necessarily being seen by health professionals; so 'people' enables a generic perspective.

The word 'care' is widely used within nursing, but less so by some other healthcare professions. Debate on the concepts of 'care' is beyond the scope of this book; for this text 'care' is intended to be interpreted in its widest sense; so, wherever 'healthcare' is available, 'care' is provided.

Terminology needs to remain flexible within its context, but ageing can conjure strong emotions. Inevitably, language surrounding ageing and healthcare provision for older people has gained emotive connotations (see Chapter 10). Where possible, language with negative or pejorative associations has been avoided.

Conclusion

This book is about, and for, the 'swampy lowlands' (Schon 1991) of practice rather than esoteric theory. So, although theoretical perspectives are presented and discussed, they are applied to practice. This book has been divided into sections to help readers find and use material. However, the life experiences of each person, and so their individual ageing, will be simultaneously affected by many or all of the factors identified (to a greater or lesser extent) in the chapters of this book. Therefore, when caring for people, a holistic, rather than a reductionist, perspective should be adopted. To help readers achieve this, key cross-references are included within the text.

There is no single or simple way to define ageing. Various mechanisms will be identified through the theories outlined in this book. There are, of course, many more theories, and, although many theories have been suggested, none is conclusively proven. Because the effects of ageing are experienced by individuals, each exposed to an accumulation of factors, no process occurs in isolation.

References

de Beauvoir S (1970) Old age. London: Penguin.

Lueckenotte AG (2000) Gerontologic nursing 2nd edn. St Louis: Mosby.

Masterson A (1999) Nursing older people in hospital. In: Redfern S J and Ross F M (eds) Nursing Older People 3rd edn. pp. 123–139. Edinburgh: Churchill Livingstone.

Schon D A (1991) The reflective practitioner. Aldershot: Arena.

Scrutton S (1992) Ageing, healthy and in control. London: Chapman and Hall.

Simons L A, McCallum J, Friedlander Y and Simons J (2000) Healthy ageing is associated with reduced and delayed disability. Age and Ageing 29 (2): 143–148.

Tinker A (1997) Older People in Modern Society 4th edn. London: Longman.

Wells T J (1980) Problems in geriatric nursing care. Edinburgh: Churchill Livingstone.

PART 1
PHYSIOLOGICAL

CHAPTER 2

Theories of biological ageing

PHILIP WOODROW

Introduction

This section of the book considers various ways in which biological function changes with age. While this section adopts a systems-based approach, each person is more than just a sum of their biological systems. Therefore, systems-based knowledge should be applied within the context of the whole person.

Throughout human history people have asked why ageing occurs, usually to try to answer how it can be reversed. While biological ageing may be delayed, so far no means has been found to reverse or even halt it, and from current perspectives it seems unlikely that such means will ever be found. Indeed, were any genuine elixir of youth to be found, presumably either human reproduction would have to end or the capacity of earth to support increasing numbers of human beings would soon become exhausted. Such a scenario would open up a mass of ethical problems.

But, while the elixir of youth remains elusive, understanding of why ageing occurs has increased significantly in recent years. There have been many theories put forward to explain ageing. Theories of biological ageing are usually divided into two groups:

- stochastic
- nonstochastic

'Stochastic' describes anything determined by a random accumulation of events, whereas nonstochastic theories involve predetermination. Stochastic theories include:

- free radicals
- error

- somatic mutation
- genetics
- cross-linking
- wear and tear.

Nonstochastic theories include:

- biological clock ('programmed ageing')
- neuroendocrine
- immunology.

The word 'stochastic' is not used further in this book. While there are too many theories for this chapter to cover either in their entirety or in depth, three of the currently more credible theories are discussed:

- biological clock
- subsequent work on apoptosis
- free radicals.

With advances in the understanding of microphysiology, the study of pathophysiology has moved away from macro body systems, such as the heart, and abstract speculation to focus on understanding how function and malfunction at cell level affects health. This is reflected in theories of biological ageing and so necessitates some discussion of cellular function, pathology and ageing, and the differences between cellular necrosis and apoptosis. No single theory has been conclusively proven; so a number of theories retain current credibility. The results of ageing are potentially confused with its causes because many of the theories listed above are the result of visual observations. But these results ignore the fact that ageing is affected by many other factors, including:

- genetic inheritance
- life experiences
- lifestyle and stress
- exercise
- smoking
- nutrition
- alcohol
- pollution

- exposure to chemicals and radiation
- poverty
- social class
- illness
- availability of health and social services.

Health and ageing can be affected by any or all of these factors, whether or not they are 'theories' of ageing. Many of these factors overlap, and exposure to them may vary during the course of a lifetime. 'Normal' physiological ageing therefore should be understood in the context of complete life experiences.

Understanding why ageing occurs, and how it can be slowed down, helps people to live as healthily as possible for as long as possible. Issues around healthy living are developed in Chapter 14.

Chapters in this section often cite chronological ages when significant physiological changes occur. Although drawn from literature, and representing a normal or average age by which such changes can be measured, problems of using chronological age are identified in the previous chapter. Each person is an individual, and physiological ageing occurs in each person at an individual rate. Having such chronological signposts can be useful to guide practice and so are cited here, but assessment and care should be individualized for each person.

Attempts to classify theories of ageing risk confusing a theory of how ageing occurs with an observation of the effects ageing has. Some theories of ageing have been induced from abstract ideas, while some have been deduced from observed symptoms. Complex interactions between body systems create a 'chicken and egg' argument, for reduced function of any system (e.g. immunity) can accelerate the reduced function, and so the ageing, of other systems.

The wear-and-tear theory

Just as a carpet in a room that is well used is likely to reach the end of its useful lifespan sooner than one in a room that is seldom used, so the wear-and-tear theory suggests that the cumulative damage sustained by cell lines (wear and tear) influences their ageing. This theory, first suggested by Weisman in 1882, fails to explain why exercise improves, rather than impairs, function (Lueckenotte 2000) and so is largely discredited. It is included here as an example of one of many theories that remained current until well into the twentieth century, when significant developments in microphysiology established the means of cellular function and so revealed the importance of cellular dysfunction in pathological processes.

Cells – the basis of life

Diseases and physical problems are experienced and diagnosed at the level of the larger, macroscopic systems of the human body. But each body system is made up of a large number of microscopic cells. The function of any tissue relies on whatever happens at cellular level. Therefore a study of physiological ageing should begin by understanding the function of human cells. A brief summary of normal cell function is given, but readers unfamiliar with this material may need to supplement their understanding from an anatomy text (such as Marieb 2001).

There are trillions of cells within the human body, with millions of different types of cells. At cellular level, life is dynamic. With conception, two cells (a sperm and an ovum) fuse. During foetal life, the number of cells will multiply enormously. The number of cells continues to increase throughout childhood. By adulthood, the rate of cell reproduction declines, but new cells continue to be needed to replace cells that are destroyed. Some body cells are able to reproduce themselves by division (mitosis); others (e.g. mature erythrocytes) are unable to divide, but are reproduced from stem cells. The lifespan of most cells is relatively short; for example, erythrocytes normally survive about 120 days. The body is thus constantly changing the complex of cells that cumulatively makes up each person. This change is a necessary part of life. To help remove cells that are dysfunctional or have fulfilled their purpose, the body has a control mechanism called 'apoptosis' (described later).

During healthy mitosis, each of the two new cells reproduces genetic codes contained within DNA (deoxyribonucleic acid). DNA division takes place before cells divide; so cell information is passed on to each succeeding generation of cells. This ensures that each succeeding generation in the cell line continues the specialized function of the cell type (for example liver sinusoid cells continue to function as liver sinusoid cells). This genetic programming within DNA may contribute towards the ageing process (Schneider 1992).

During cell reproduction significant changes can occur. Sometimes mutations occur (for example, cancerous cells, which usually lose any specialist nature or function). Mitosis of mutated cells is likely to produce similarly mutated cells. So cell health must be considered not in terms of the lifespan of a single cell but in the 'cell line' – all succeeding generations of similar cells that derive from a cell type. Cell mutation may just result from chance, or be caused by toxic substances (e.g. radiation).

The rate of cell reproduction tends to decline with age. As the length of cell life remains unchanged, cell numbers decline, resulting in tissue atrophy or loss. In some tissues, living cells are replaced by inert substances (e.g. plaques in blood vessels) or different kinds of tissue (e.g. muscle replaced by adipose tissue). Changes inevitably alter tissue function. However, the extent and nature of functional change varies greatly between different tissues. Various tissue and function changes are discussed in later chapters. Theories of biological ageing attempt to explain why reproduction rates decline.

Cells survive in a delicate internal environment. The delicate internal environment is protected by the cell membrane. Cell membranes are semi-permeable. The transfer of most fluids and solutes across cell membranes is actively regulated by various 'pumps', of which the sodium/potassium pump is probably the best known. At rest, extracellular levels of sodium (about 140 mmol per litre) and potassium (about 4 mmol per litre) are approximately reversed in intracellular fluid (i.e. sodium about 14 mmol/litre, potassium about 140 mmol/litre, (Guyton and Hall 2000).

In health, cell membranes are able to respond rapidly to restore homeostasis. But damaged membranes (e.g. from hypoxia) are less effective at maintaining control between the internal and external environments of the body. Damaged membranes become more leaky, facilitating movement of water, sodium and calcium into the cell. Sodium and water cause the cell to swell (intracellular oedema), which causes further mechanical damage to, and possible rupture of, the cell membrane. Damaged membranes release various intracellular enzymes and chemicals. Myocardial infarction can be diagnosed by the levels of creatine kinase (CK) or troponin in the blood. Other enzymes released from damaged cells can cause a range of symptoms and tissue damage throughout the body.

The balance of each cell's internal environment is maintained by various parts of the cell itself. For example, cells contain organelles called *mitochondria*, which use fuels such as sugars and fats to produce adenosine triphosphate (ATP), the energy needed by the cell to live. ATP production releases waste products of water, carbon dioxide and metabolic acids. All these waste products can transfer easily across the cell membrane and so be removed by the blood stream. Energy production also releases some free radicals; the effects of free radicals are discussed later in this chapter, as this has formed one theory of biological ageing.

Cell damage

Cell damage can be caused by:

- deficiency
- intoxication
- trauma.

Deficiency of any substance needed for the cell to function will cause cell damage. Cells need oxygen and nutrients. Inadequate oxygen (e.g. poor perfusion) causes cell metabolism to change from aerobic (oxygen-based) to anaerobic (non-oxygen-based). Anaerobic metabolism is very inefficient, producing relatively little energy. Aerobic metabolism produces 38 ATP molecules from each gram of glucose, whereas anaerobic metabolism produces only two (Nathan and Singer 1999). Because anaerobic metabolism produces so little energy per gram of glucose, metabolic rate is greatly increased in a compensatory attempt to sustain ATP production. This results in far greater quantities of waste products, which, if not removed (for example during low-perfusion states such as shock), further alter the intracellular and extracellular environments, causing further cell damage.

In the absence of glucose, mitochondria will use fats to generate energy. But, like anaerobic metabolism, fats produce a relatively large amount of waste. Hence the metabolic acidosis and other problems seen during a diabetic crisis (e.g. diabetic ketoacidosis).

Intoxication is caused by any substance that interferes with cell function. Toxins may be exogenous (from outside the body) or endogenous (produced by the body). Exogenous toxins may be biological (e.g. bacteria) or non-biological (e.g. chemicals such as carbon tetrachloride, which is used in dry cleaning). Endogenous toxins include free (gas) radicals, tumour necrosis factor alpha and interleukins, all chemicals that are release by damaged cells.

Trauma – direct physical injury to the cell – is caused by mechanical pressure, either from inside or outside the cell. A virus can invade a cell, becoming a parasite multiplying within the cell. Viral multiplication will eventually cause the cell membrane to rupture, releasing parasites into neighbouring cells. Cell trauma may be caused by exposing the cell to an altered environment (e.g. hyperthermia, hypothermia and radiation) or from increased pressure from surrounding tissues (e.g. tumours). Pressure sores are a visible result of external mechanical pressure on superficial tissue.

Pathological problems may be caused by extensive damage of any kind to a cell within the body, including bacteria. So damage to bacterial cell membranes from the body's own defence mechanisms (e.g. white blood cells) or from antibiotics can release many of the powerful chemical mediators mentioned above. For example, Gram-negative bacteria contain endotoxin that, with other chemical mediators, causes many of the symptoms of infection. During infection, some of the body's own cells will also be damaged, releasing various powerful chemical mediators. One of these, interleukin 1, causes pyrexia and various other responses.

Cell death

Cell death can be caused by:

- necrosis
- apoptosis.

Necrosis is an inflammatory process, causing cells to swell. Swelling of cells damages their membranes, allowing contents from the cell to leak into extracellular fluid. This process, which has been described above, causes the systemic release of powerful chemicals and underlies many acute disease processes (e.g. sepsis). Apoptosis, sometimes called 'programmed cell death', is currently viewed as a major cause of ageing.

Apoptosis

Apoptosis is a homeostatic mechanism used in health to eliminate unwanted cells from the body. For example, the body contains various safeguards against cell mutation and invasion by foreign organisms, such as the T-lymphocytes (part of the immune system). Few 2%-3%, (Hong 1992) of the T-lymphoblasts survive to maturation, most being selectively destroyed. This selection process normally prevents lymphocytes, which are released, from attacking the body's own tissue (Abbas et al 1994). Failure of this selection process leads to autoimmunity. Autoimmunity can cause various disease processes, including arthritis.

Although originating in bone marrow, T-lymphoblasts migrate to the thymus gland during an early stage of their development. Children have relatively large thymus glands, but following puberty the gland becomes virtually undetectable (Abbas et al 1994), being replaced by adipose and connective tissue (Marieb 2001). T-lymphocytes can survive more than twenty years, and maturation does continue throughout life (Abbas et al 1994), possibly in other, as-yet-undetected, maturation sites. However, immune function does decline with age, partly due to decreased numbers of circulating lymphocytes. For example, immunity and immunodeficiency have in the past been included among theories of ageing. But, although immunity does usually decline with age, this decline appears to be a symptom, rather than a cause, of ageing.

Apoptosis signals expressed on the outer membranes of cells will initiate phagocytosis (Savill 1997). During apoptosis, DNA (the genetic code of the cell) is broken (Honig and Rosenberg 2000). However, the membrane remains intact; so, in contrast to necrosis, intracellular enzymes remain within the cell (Savill 1997). Therefore, there is no significant injury to, or inflammation of, other tissues (Haslett 1997).

Deficiencies in apoptosis (either too much or too little) may contribute to persistent inflammatory and immune diseases (Savill 1997, Ekert and Vaux 1997), such as arthritis. At present, too little is known about specific receptors to target them with drugs, but, theoretically, apoptosis could be induced as a means of treating some disease processes (Haslett 1997).

The biological clock

The past two centuries have seen significant increases in life expectancy (at birth) for people living in Western countries. However, although premature mortality has been reduced, there has been relatively little increase in the maximum age at which the oldest people die (Tinker 1997); the extreme limit of human life appears to be about 120 years (Lueckenotte 2000), although few people survive for a century. This suggests that there may be some finite limit to human life. It has been speculated that this upper limit could be genetically programmed.

Some genetic research in the twentieth century suggested that in ideal situations human cells, or human cell lines, could be immortal. However, such research used abnormal (cancerous) cells, which do not reproduce normally (Hayflick 1985). Culturing human fibroblasts in a laboratory setting, Hayflick (1985) found that the mitosis of normal human embryonic cells was limited to about 50 cell divisions. From this evidence, Hayflick concluded that the number of times cells would divide before dying was finite, and therefore life was effectively controlled by a 'chronometer or pacemaker within all normal cells' (Hayflick 1985 p. 21), and that age-related changes occurred as a result of a loss of function at the cellular level.

In 1994 a substance called *telomerase* was discovered. Telomerase is an enzyme that protects telomeres (part of the chromosome) from degrading (Marieb 2001). Telomerase therefore appears to confer immortality.

Telomerase is almost always found in cancer cells but seldom, or in very small amounts, in other cells (Marieb 2001). This would explain why lines of cancer cells are able to be 'immortalized' in laboratory conditions.

Free radical theory

Atoms that are unstable on their own normally exist in pairs. For example, oxygen (O) normally exists as a paired molecule (O_2). A single oxygen atom (O) is therefore highly unstable and reactive and so will rapidly initiate a chemical reaction to try to form a more stable combination. These highly reactive, unstable atoms are called 'free radicals', or sometimes just 'radicals'. A free radical is a molecule with one or more unpaired electrons in its outer orbit. Although there are many types of radicals, oxygen radicals, including the superoxide combinations (e.g. O_3), appear to be the most pathological within the human body.

The lifespan of a single radical atom is very brief – a number of microseconds (Davidson and Boom 1995). Being unstable, they readily react with other molecules to form a further molecule. If two oxygen radicals react, a stable oxygen molecule will be formed (O_2), but, if one radical reacts with a non-radical, another radical is likely to be produced. This sequence of unstable reactions is often thousands of 'generations' (combinations) long (Davidson and Boom, 1995). Large numbers of chemical reactions occurring within body cells are likely to cause damage, a process also known as 'autocatalysis'. Cell membranes are particularly susceptible to damage from free radicals (Nowak and Handford 1996). Free radicals may therefore cause cell-related changes responsible for the ageing process.

Intracellular energy production inevitably produces some free radicals. Free radical production is significantly increased by exposure to ionizing radiation (e.g. excessive sunlight, X-rays) (Nowak and Handford 1996). The body uses a number of free radical scavengers to destroy these potentially dangerous chemicals and restore homeostasis. Some free radical scavengers are produced within the body (e.g. N-acetylcysteine, cytosolic superoxide dismutase and albumin) and some are absorbed from foods (such as vitamins C and E). As the most problematic free radical is usually oxygen, free-radical scavengers are often called 'antioxidants'. Diets of older people are often poorer than those of younger people, and their digestion and absorption of nutrients is often reduced. So the number and effect of free radical scavengers is likely to be poorer. However, in addition to their presence in various foods, many free radical scavengers (especially vitamins C and E) can be taken as vitamin supplement tablets (or injections). Many are available as over-the-counter medicines, some labelled as 'antioxidants', while others are contained in vitamin combinations or sold as individual chemicals (e.g. vitamin E). Although vitamins have relatively few side effects, people should seek pharmaceutical advice about doses and possible interactions with any other medicines they are taking. A healthy diet is therefore usually a safer option than taking unprescribed tablet supplements.

Factors affecting ageing

Although theories, such as those described above, suggest possible explanations for the biological basis of ageing, the complex interactions of physiological, psychological and social factors cannot be separated as neatly in life as they can in a laboratory or on paper. Ageing is influenced by a range of factors that can accelerate or slow down the process. People in the higher levels of the Registrar General's social-classification scheme have a higher life and health expectancy (Black et al 1982), a gap that has widened, rather than narrowed, since the Black Report was first published (Goldblatt and Whitehead 2000). While gender and genetic inheritance can affect ageing and the process of a disease, this genetic inheritance is not class related. Clearly, life and health expectancy derive from factors that individuals are exposed to throughout their lives. Various factors that affect ageing will be identified further in subsequent chapters.

Homeostasis

Cell health relies on maintenance of the delicate internal balance. When this balance is disrupted, the body uses various controls and responses, most mediated through the autonomic nervous system, to restore the balance.

Temperature regulation provides a good illustration of homeostasis. Body temperature is controlled by the pituitary gland, which receives information from both peripheral-temperature (touch) receptors in the skin and receptors in the pituitary gland itself, which sense the temperature of blood in the brain. When the pituitary gland identifies excessive body heat, it initiates autonomic nerve signals to dilate blood vessels and increase sweat production. Both of these increase heat loss. Low body temperature stimulates vasoconstriction of peripheral blood vessels, which conserves heat, and causes shivering, which produces heat.

In health, the pituitary gland maintains body temperature within a narrow range; although 'normal' varies between individuals, most people have a normal temperature of about 36°C–37°C. However, diseases, such as infection, can cause the pituitary gland (or any other homeostatic mechanism) to malfunction, resulting in it attempting to 'restore' the body to an abnormally high temperature.

Age-related changes affect homeostasis. For example, peripheral-temperature receptors or nerve conduction may be less effective, causing people to become less sensitive to cold weather. Together with other factors, such as reduced metabolism causing less heat to be produced, and poverty making them reluctant to turn on heating in their homes, this can expose them to hypothermia.

A cure for ageing?

Implicit in attempts to explain how physiological ageing occurs is a wish to control, and perhaps reverse, it. While the 'elixir of youth' remains elusive, current therapies, such as hormone replacement therapy or antioxidants, are widely available. Where these bring benefits, and they often do, their use is justified. However, there is a danger that age and ageing are viewed as diseases that need to be cured, or at least treated (Illich 1976). Ageing is a natural process, and old age is not a disease. Ill health is more likely to occur with old age, and ill health should be treated. Where any cure is impossible, unethical or unkind, the person should be offered whatever control is in their best interests (e.g. pain control). However, where age-related changes do not cause actual or potential problems to the individual, no attempt should normally be made to reverse them. Most age-related changes do not cause problems. So the potentially negative lists of decline that appear in this section of the book should be read in the context of perspectives of health rather than disease.

Conclusion

Many theories have been put forward to try to explain why ageing occurs. Although no one theory has yet been conclusively proven, this chapter summarizes the theories that currently seem to be the most reliable. With research and laboratory evidence accumulating, each current theory has considerable supporting evidence, unlike some earlier theories. Knowledge of cell function increased greatly in the latter half of the twentieth century, much subsequent work being based on Hayflick's pioneering studies. This knowledge has shifted the focus of theories from macroscopic-whole-body-system perspectives to the microscopic, and from metaphysical speculation to laboratory-tested knowledge. However, there is still much that remains unknown, including the fundamental question of *why* ageing occurs.

While the study of why ageing occurs may lead to worthwhile medical treatments, for healthcare workers the important question is not why ageing has occurred but how ageing affects each person they work with. Understanding the causes of physiological ageing should help health professionals find ways to help each individual minimize or reverse any further loss of function. This knowledge should not be used to blame the individual for their past or present choice of lifestyle, however much those choices may have hastened their physiological ageing. So, for example, the diabetic with an unhealthy diet should be offered health advice, but not criticism. The right of each individual to choose their lifestyle should be respected.

The remaining chapters in this section will outline the main physiological effects of normal ageing, as well as pathophysiological (abnormal ageing) changes. Although pathological problems originate at the cellular level, by the time symptoms occur, extensive cellular dysfunction has resulted in the whole system being affected. The remaining chapters in this section will therefore discuss system decline and failure, together with disease processes. This potentially negative perspective should be considered in the context of the continuing ability of most systems to maintain adequate levels of function, and the ability of most old people to lead 'healthy' lives. Staff working with older people can apply their knowledge of physiological ageing to explore and develop ways to maintain optimal quality of life for their clients. Ageing is a process, not a disease. Ageing, and living, healthily is developed further in Chapter 14.

References

Abbas A K, Lichtman A H, Pober J S (1994) Cellular and Molecular Immunology. 2nd edn. Philadelphia: W B Saunders.

Black D, Morris J N, Smith C and Townsend P (1982) Inequalities in Health. London: Penguin.

Davidson J A H and Boom S J (1995) The significance of free radicals. British Journal of Intensive Care 5 (5): 150–155 + 5 (6): 185–193.

Ekert P G and Vaux D L (1997) Apoptosis and the immune system. British Medical Bulletin 53 (3): 591-603.

Goldblatt P and Whitehead M (2000) Inequalities in health – development and change. Population Trends, Summer 14–19.

Guyton A C and Hall J E (2000) Textbook of Medical Physiology. 10th edn. Philadelphia: WB Saunders Company.

Haslett C (1997) Granulocyte apoptosis and inflammatory disease. British Medical Bulletin. 53 (3): 669–683.

Hayflick L (1985) The cell biology of ageing. Clinical Geriatric Medicine 1 (1): 15–27.

Hong R (1992) Structure and function of the immune system. In: Fuhrman BP and Zimmerman J J (eds) Pediatric Critical Care pp. 907–916. St Louis: Mosby.

Honig L S and Rosenberg R N (2000) Apoptosis and neurologic disease. American Journal of Medicine 108 (4): 317–330.

Illich I (1976) Limits to Medicine London: Penguin.

Lueckenotte A G (2000) Gerontologic Nursing 2nd edn. St Louis: Mosby.

Marieb E N (2001) Human Anatomy and Physiology 5th edn. San Francisco: Benjamin/Cummings Publishing Company Inc.

Nathan A T and Singer M (1999) The oxygen trail: tissue oxygenation. British Medical Bulletin 55 (1): 96–108.

Nowak T J and Handford A G (1996) Essentials of Pathophysiology. Iowa: Wm C Brown Publishers.

Savill J (1997) Recognition and phagocytosis of cells undergoing apoptosis. British Medical Bulletin 53 (3): 491–508.

Schneider E (1992) Biological theories of aging. Generations 16 (4): 7–11.

Tinker A (1997) Older People in Modern Society 4th edn. London: Longman.

CHAPTER 3

Skin, muscles and bones

PHILIP WOODROW

Introduction

This chapter illustrates the effects of ageing on skin, muscle and bone function. Although impaired function of these parts of the body affects health, skin (including hair) is also highly visible. Therefore changes to skin and hair also affect the person's self-image. While skin bears the marks of our life and lifestyle, physiological changes occurring just below the skin's surface can have significant effects on health. These subcutaneous changes are also explored in this chapter.

The section on skin includes discussion of pressure sores (decubitus ulcers). The section on muscles is shorter, but is included to identify a major factor in age-related loss of strength. Discussion of bone ageing includes sections on teeth and on arthritis. Falls, which are a major problem for many older people, are briefly discussed.

Skin

Structure

The skin is more than just a container for the body; it has a complex series of functions (see Table 3.1) that can too often be overlooked until problems occur. Skin has two layers: the *epidermis* and the *dermis*.

The epidermis, forming the outer layer, is mainly dead epithelial cells. These dead cells provide valuable protection against the knocks, bumps and shearing forces that skin surfaces are inevitably exposed to. Each day millions of epidermal cells will be lost. Skin surfaces also provide a barrier between external and internal environments, preventing invasion of body tissue by micro-organisms (bacteria, viruses) in the atmosphere or on skin surfaces. Damage to the skin's surface (e.g. surgical wounds, pressure

Table 3.1: Functions of the skin

- protection
- tissue repair
- touch
- temperature regulation
- excretion

sores) provides a means of entry for environmental or skin-surface organisms.

The dermis is mostly fibrous connective tissue. Unlike the epidermis, it is living tissue. Most skin functions, other than protection, originate in the dermis. The dermal layer contains blood vessels, nerves, hair follicle roots, sweat glands, sebaceous glands and sensory receptors (touch, temperature, pain). Dermal papillae project into the epidermis, connecting the two layers together.

The dermis has two layers, a superficial papillary layer and a deeper reticular layer. The reticular layer forms about 80% of dermal tissue (Marieb 2001) and contains collagen fibres. Collagen is tough and so provides protection against trauma. It also binds water and so keeps skin hydrated (Marieb 2001). Collagen reduces by about 1 per cent each year, making skin weaker and so more prone to tearing (Schofield 1999). Remaining collagen cross-links reduce the elasticity of the skin and make it wrinkled (Schofield 1999).

Below the dermis (so, below the skin) is the hypodermis, a layer of adipose tissue. The hypodermis anchors the dermis to underlying tissue while remaining flexible, and provides heat insulation (Marieb 2001).

Sweat

The skin contains more than two and a half million sweat (sudoriferous) glands, which normally secrete about 500 millilitres of sweat each day (Marieb 2001). There are two main types of sweat gland:

- eccrine
- apocrine.

Apocrine glands, found mainly in axillar and ano-genital areas, also secrete fats and proteins. Metabolism of this fat and protein by skin-surface bacteria causes body odour (Marieb 2001).

Sweat is mainly (99%) water (Marieb 2001). Even in cool conditions, about 10% of insensible water loss occurs through skin (Clancy and

McVicar 1995). Sweat also contains salts, vitamin C, antibodies, urea, uric acid, ammonia and lactic acid (Marieb 2001). Compared to kidneys, skin has only a limited role in regulating fluid balance, but it is significant enough to have been used in Roman times for dialysis (hot bathing increases the skin's urea loss). Although sweat is commonly viewed as a nuisance, and something to be suppressed with antiperspirants, it:

- controls body temperature
- excretes waste products
- provides immunity.

Increased body temperature increases sweat production. This is a homeo-static mechanism, increasing heat loss by evaporation of the water in sweat. Up to 12 litres of sweat can be lost daily (Marieb 2001). Prolonged, profuse sweating can cause serious dehydration. Sweat also contains sodium chloride; so excessive sweating may also cause hyponatraemia.

Sebaceous glands

Sebaceous glands are found everywhere in the skin except for palms of hands and soles of feet (Marieb 2001). They secrete sebum, a thick oily substance that softens and lubricates hair and skin. Most sebum is secreted into hair follicles, hence potential problems with 'oily' hair. Sebum also contains antibacterial substances, providing protecting against invasion by skin-surface bacteria.

Before puberty, sebaceous glands are relatively inactive, but during puberty androgens and, to a lesser extent, other hormones significantly increase sebum production (Marieb 2001). So adolescents, especially boys, often develop acne and blackheads (Wong et al 1999).

Ageing

With age, skin function declines. In younger people, the epidermis is renewed every 20 days, but renewal time increases by one-third after the age of 50 (Schofield 1999), and the epidermis flattens (Herbert 1999). Sutures may therefore need to remain longer in older skin. Epidermal and dermal layers of skin may peel apart more easily, making older people more prone to pressure sores from shearing, such as being dragged over a surface (Herbert 1999).

With age, dermal cells decline both in number and function. There are fewer skin capillaries and so the skin is supplied with less oxygen, nutrients and fluids (Herbert 1999). Re-epithelization takes approximately twice as long for a 75-year-old as for a 25-year-old. So any wounds (trauma, surgery or pressure sores) will take longer to heal. Age-related reduction in hormone production also reduces sebum production (Marieb 2001), making skin and hair dryer, more brittle, itchy, wrinkled and prone to tearing (cuts and sores). Broken nails can be particularly irritating for people.

When cutaneous drugs are used, reduced numbers of capillaries result in the slower absorption of any cutaneous drugs (Herbert 1999). Cutaneous drugs include not only glyceryl trinitrate (GTN) or nicotine patches but also any 'essential' oils used for massage.

As sensory-nerve function is reduced, older people are less able to feel touch, pain or temperature (Herbert 1999). This exposes them to greater risks from cuts, burns or hypothermia.

Many genetic and environmental factors affect skin, and so skin ageing. Most changes are irreversible, but care of the skin can slow its ageing. Skin is particularly sensitive to activation of enzymes by the sun's ultraviolet rays; so shielding the skin from sunlight slows skin ageing (Marieb 2001). Other care, such as a well-balanced diet and good skin hygiene, may also restrict the skin from ageing.

Pressure sores

Ten percent of hospitalized patients develop pressure sores, most occurring in patients aged over 70 (Reid and Morison 1994). Waterlow (1995) divides causes of pressure-sore formation between intrinsic (factors within the body) and extrinsic (factors from outside). Intrinsic factors cited by Waterlow are:

- ageing
- malnutrition
- dehydration
- incontinence
- medical condition
- medication.

Extrinsic factors cited are:

- pressure
- shearing
- friction.

Capillaries remove waste products of cellular metabolism (e.g. lactic acid). Metabolic rate slows with age, but removal of waste products also reduces; so toxic waste products of metabolism may accumulate in peripheral tissues, increasing the risk of skin breakdown (Waterlow 1995). Capillaries also supply oxygen, nutrients and other factors needed for both normal function and tissue repair. Therefore tissue without an adequate capillary supply will die. A pressure sore is a localized area of tissue necrosis (Reid and Morison 1994).

For capillaries to perfuse an area, the pressure in a blood vessel must be greater than the pressure of tissue resistance. So, where an area of skin is pressed against a bed mattress, chair or anything else creating extrinsic pressure, the capillary pressure needs to be greater than the extrinsic pressure in order to perfuse the tissue.

Blood pressure progressively reduces as blood travels through the cardiovascular system. Capillary pressures are as variable as arterial pressures, but they are also considerably lower, ranging between 18 and 35 mmHg (Dealey 1992).

Ischaemia prevents the removal of waste products. The causes of ischaemia may be acute (e.g. shock, major haemorrhage) or chronic (e.g. peripheral vascular disease). The accumulation of waste products, including acids produced through metabolism, progressive tissue hypoxia and undernourishment results in cell death and further tissue damage. This may initially be seen as a first-grade pressure sore (redness in skin). Without oxygen and nutrients needed for repair, the breakdown of skin surfaces is likely to follow. Excessively moist or dry skin is likely to break down more rapidly; so lubricating dry skin (e.g. with aqueous cream) can reduce the risk of ulceration.

Prevention

A rational approach to pressure-sore prevention needs to recognize what can and cannot be changed. Gravity, for example, cannot realistically be changed. But the area on which each patient is resting can be changed. So, rather than concentrating gravity through a small area, spreading that force over a larger area may prevent pressure sores.

Pressure-relieving mattresses and aids exerting constant pressures above capillary-occlusion pressure are unlikely to be effective. From the above figures, extrinsic pressures below 25 mmHg should be safe for most people. In-house aids are usually too inaccurate to be recommended, especially when so many commercially available mattresses and aids are available. Unless extrinsic pressure from in-house aids can be measured, they raise problems around professional accountability and potential litigation. For example, water-filled gloves are usually overfilled with water, so exerting pressures greater than 25 mmHg; being concave, they also concentrate this high pressure on a small area.

Some intrinsic factors identified by Waterlow, such as ageing, cannot be reversed. But good nutrition and continence can be promoted. Protein loss in the exudate from an open sore and the energy cost of healing can increase nutritional needs by 1000 kcal each day. In addition to providing comfort and dignity, faecal continence should be promoted to prevent skin damage from acids in faeces (Lowry 1995). Mattresses allowing more circulation of air will help remove excessive skin moisture (from incontinence, wound exudate, or skin secretions), although they should not be used as a substitute for washes.

In addition to the human cost of suffering caused by pressure sores, any negligence may result in litigation. Tingle (1997) cites litigation costs ranging between £4,500 and £12,500. Health professionals are individually accountable for their actions and so have a professional duty to ensure that practice is based on sound evidence.

Hair

Hair growth slows after the fourth decade, with less than a third of hair follicles remaining by the fifth decade (Marieb 2001). Loss of hair is often more marked in men, especially on the scalp, largely due to androgens. Although scalp hair on women thins, a greater threat to their body image can be from post-menopausal growth of facial hair, especially a faint 'moustache'. Some drugs, such as steroids, increase the growth of facial hair.

Hair colour results from pigmentation by melanocytes. As melanin production declines, air bubbles increasingly fill hair shafts, making hair grey or white (Marieb 2001). 'Greying' is a highly visible sign and so can also threaten the patient's self-image.

Muscles

Much of the body is muscle. Muscle is protein and enables movement. But muscle also stores many substances. Muscle mass is increased during anabolism and broken down during catabolism.

The main anabolic hormone is the male hormone testosterone, hence its (mis)use as an anabolic steroid to improve sporting performance. Most testosterone is produced in the testes; although neither 'male' nor 'female' hormones are exclusively gender-specific, and small amounts of both are produced in the adrenal glands regardless of gender. Testosterone causes most adult men to have more muscle mass and weight than most adult women. Gender differences in muscle mass and strength become especially noticeable among older people (Hyatt et al 1990) although age-related reduction in testosterone production results in replacement of muscle mass with adipose tissue.

Much of the body's water is contained in its muscle tissue; so, as muscle mass is replaced by fat (which repels water), total body water is reduced. This makes older people more prone to dehydration. Muscle protein is also a potential fuel source, so during starvation, including extended pre-operative fasting, older people are more likely to develop complications.

Muscle tone atrophies steadily from the age of 30 (Schofield 1999), muscle mass declines from an average 24 kg to 13 kg and fat increases from an average 15 kg to 25 kg between the ages of 25 and 75 (Devlin 2000). By the age of 80, muscle strength has decreased by at least 30 per cent (Hyatt et al 1990). Older people therefore often have significant loss of muscle strength. Muscle weakness contributes to the risk of falls and complications from limited mobility. Recovery from illness may be slowed by respiratory-muscle weakness. This weakness can impair many activities of living, ranging from mobility to continence. The effect on activities of living is illustrated below by bowel function. Constipation, a frequent complication of bowel dysfunction, is discussed in chapter 5.

Falls

Falls are the most common type of accident bringing people aged over 65 years old into accident and emergency departments (Bowling and Grant 1992), affecting 28–35% of people over 65 (living in the community) and more than 40% of people over 75 (Davies and Kenny 1996). Falls are the sixth-largest cause of death in older people (Gray and Hildebrand 2000). Gray and Hildebrand suggest that falls may result from:

- diseases (e.g. Parkinson's Disease)
- complications of treatment (especially cardiac drugs such as beta-blockers)
- risk factors of ageing (e.g. visual loss).

While some falls cause little more than discomfort and inconvenience, others may result in hospitalization, bed rest or surgery.

An instinctive reaction when falling is to stretch out our arms to break the fall. But brittle older bones are more likely to break; the radius bone that connects the arm with the hand is especially likely to break (*Colles' fracture*). The incidence of Colles' fractures is especially high in women aged over 50 (Holt 2000) due to the effects of post-menopausal osteoporosis.

Bowel dysfunction

The colon is surrounded by muscle. Normal peristalsis moves faecal matter through the colon over a period of 12–24 hours. Colonic muscle suffers similar atrophy to other muscles; so with age peristalsis becomes weaker. Straining at stool increases the pressure on the muscle walls, potentially causing damage such as diverticula (Herbert 1999).

Ageing does not in itself reduce gut motility or bowel frequency (Norton 1996; Koch and Hudson 2000), although colonic muscle tone is reduced. Constipation is likely to be caused by one or more of the following:

- poor diet (low fibre)
- laxative abuse (reducing muscle tone)
- dehydration (insufficient fluid intake)
- limited mobility.

Many other factors can contribute to constipation. Older people are often exposed to more than one factor; so those helping people suffering from constipation should assess which factors are significant and which ones can be treated.

Bones

Skeletons and bones found in most anatomy classrooms illustrate their shape but can give false impressions of living physiology. Bone inside living people is itself a living substance and, like any other body tissue, is constantly changing and being replaced. At birth, the overall shape of human skeleton is complete, but bones grow and develop further throughout childhood. During adult life, the shape of bones does not significantly change (unless they are fractured or undergo surgery), but ageing does affect bones in various ways. Each week 5–7% of bone mass is recycled, although from the fourth decade destruction of bone tissue exceeds replacement, resulting in an overall reduction in bone mass (Marieb 2001). Loss of bone mass contributes to age-related loss of height, which, from about 40 years of age, reduces by about 1.5 centimetres every 20 years (Schofield 1999).

The most obvious function of the skeletal system is to provide the shape of the body to enable people to stand upright. But bones also have a number of other functions, including:

- erythrocyte production
- immunity (leucocyte and lymphocyte production)
- storage (especially of calcium).

All of these functions are affected by a reduction in bone mass.

Bone is made mainly of calcium. The average adult human body contains 1200–1400 grams of calcium, 99% of which is stored within bone (Marieb 2001). Calcium is also needed elsewhere in the body, especially for muscle contraction (cardiac and skeletal). Muscular work relies on the remaining 1% of body calcium in the bloodstream. Blood calcium is regulated by the parathyroid hormone parathormone; therefore, hyperparathyroidism causes hypercalcaemia, while hypoparathyroidism causes hypocalcaemia (Solomon et al 1990). But, with age, the calcium stores in bone are depleted more quickly than they are replaced, resulting in osteoporosis and hypocalcaemia. Hypocalcaemia impairs muscle function.

Bone calcium provides a store for blood calcium. Without calcium, normal muscle movement and control would not be possible. Calcium is also used for clotting (e.g. healing of pressure sores). So, the bone stores calcium, which the body can withdraw when needed and replace when surplus is available.

Growth

Bone growth (including replacement of bone cells) is controlled by various hormones, including thyroid hormones (T3, T4), parathyroid hormones and testosterone. But a range of nutrients is also needed for bone growth. Vitamin D is needed for calcium to be absorbed (Marieb 2001). Other nutrients needed include vitamins A and C and a number of other minerals, including phosphorus, magnesium and manganese (Marieb 2001). A deficiency of any nutrients impairs bone repair. For example, insufficient calcium (or vitamin D) results in the production of normal bone cells, but insufficient deposition of calcium salts. This causes bones to become soft (osteomalacia, or – in children – rickets), and painful when any weight is placed on them (Marieb 2001). However, it should be remembered that older people may be malnourished for a range of physiological, social, financial or other reasons.

Ageing

Bone weakness and calcium loss are multi-factorial. The diets of older people often lack sufficient calcium to meet anatomic needs, while the gut's ability to absorb calcium declines with age (Herbert 1999); so the body draws on its lifetime's savings of calcium in its bones. Dieticians can offer useful advice to optimize dietary calcium. However, any leaching of calcium from the bone almost inevitably exceeds the body's ability to absorb calcium. Vitamin D helps prevent age-related calcium loss, which in turn reduces the rate of bone loss, but the diets of many older people are low in vitamin D (Devlin 2000).

The ageing of bone is also affected by a number of other factors. Many of these cause abnormal ageing, resulting in disease. For example, a number of deficiencies has been identified in people suffering from arthritis. Low levels of vitamins A, E and beta-carotene have been found in those suffering from arthritis (Comstock et al 1997). Vitamin E is an anti-oxidant that helps prevent some of the tissue damage caused by free oxygen radicals. Comstock et al speculate that low levels of vitamin E and other antioxidants may enable free radicals to cause the joint damage seen in arthritis. Similarly, inadequate apoptosis and the presence of a range of cytokines, including tumour necrosis factor alpha and interleukin 1 beta, have been identified with rheumatoid arthritis (Tak and Bresnihan 2000). Whether or not these are causes or results of a pathological process, their identification has led to hopes that new drugs and other therapies may be developed.

Spinal changes

The spine is a combination of a large number of bones:

- 7 cervical
- 12 thoracic
- 5 lumbar
- 5 sacrum (fused)
- 4 coccyx (fused).

A small minority of people (about 5%) have different numbers of verte-brae (Marieb 2001).

Between each (unfused) vertebra is a spinal disc. These discs provide a cushion between vertebrae, preventing damage to bones from vigorous movement (e.g. running). Discs also help make the spine more flexible, allowing the body to twist in various directions. Spinal discs account for about one-quarter of the height of the spinal column (Marieb 2001).

In the middle to later years of life spinal discs become thinner, less well hydrated and less elastic (Marieb 2001). Risks of disc herniation increase with age (Marieb 2001); displacement or herniation of spinal discs ('slipped disc') is usually extremely painful and potentially dangerous.

The spinal column is the only part of the skeleton connecting the pelvis to the head and arms. Therefore any change in the spinal column will affect posture. Women are especially susceptible to bone loss from the spine (Herbert 1999). With age, the spine tends to curve; this curvature becomes especially marked in the thoracic spine (Marieb 2001). As the spine becomes increasingly curved, *kyphosis* develops. There are other changes that can occur to the spinal column's (and body's) shape, such as *scoliosis* (curving to one side) and *lordosis* (the lumbar spine becomes more concave, causing the person to stoop forward). Spine curvature also contributes to a loss of height.

When the body's centre of gravity changes, people attempt (usually subconsciously) to alter their posture to restore their centre of gravity through their spine. With prolonged/permanent changes of posture, people may develop different (often apparently awkward) ways of standing and walking.

Osteoporosis

Osteoporosis, a weakening of the bone due to calcium loss, is a condition particularly associated with post-menopausal women, although incidence is increasing among men and younger women (Turner 2000). Citing statistics from the early 1980s, Quantock and Benyon (1994) suggest osteoporosis affects 50% of women over 70. At eighteen years of age women have on average 20% less bone than men (Herbert 1999) and so begin adult life with smaller calcium stores than men. Calcium loss from bones is particularly rapid in the five to ten years following menopause (Herbert 1999), owing to a reduced production of hormones.

Osteoporosis increases the risk of fractures and prolongs healing. In the UK osteoporosis causes more than 200,000 fractures every year in people over 50 (Wood 2000). Of those with osteoporosis, 15% will fracture a hip, and 24% of these will die as a result (usually indirectly) of the fracture (Quantock and Benyon 1994), although oestrogen-replacement therapy begun at menopause reduces the number of osteoporosis-related fractures by at least half (Lufkin et al 1992). Fractured bones may result in a potentially fatal fat embolus, although fortunately this complication is relatively rare, occurring in 0.5–2% of long bone fractures and nearly 1%

of multiple fractures (Pellegrini and Evarts 1991). Typically, younger (age 55+) people with osteoporosis suffer wrist fractures, while older (75+) people are more likely to suffer hip fractures (Wood 2000). A fractured hip will usually necessitate bed rest or other forms of treatment limiting mobility. With other body functions reduced by ageing, older people with fractures are at greater risk of developing complications, such as potentially fatal chest infections.

Hormone replacement therapy reduces the rate of bone loss and so can reduce the risk of fractures by 50–60% (Wood 2000). Oestrogen-replacement therapy is most effective when begun within five years of the menopause, and taken for more than ten years (Cauley et al 1995), although even once osteoporosis has developed oestrogen can reduce the risk of fractures (Lufkin et al 1992). But many older women underwent menopause before the widespread availability of hormone replacement therapy, or may not be receiving it for a variety of other reasons, including concerns about breast cancer with long-term use (Sahota and Masud 1999). For these women, osteoporosis and its many complications will continue to present problems for the foreseeable future. At present, osteoporosis rates are increasing disproportionately to the ageing of the UK population (Turner 2000).

The risks of developing osteoporosis later in life can be reduced by increasing bone mass, which will increase calcium stores. The years when bone density formation reaches its peak are 20–25 years of age for spongy bones and 35–40 for long bones; so ensuring sufficient dietary calcium in younger adult life will maximize calcium stores within the skeletal system (Marieb 2001). Weight-bearing exercise (during all stages of life) also helps to build bone tissue (Marieb 2001). However, the decreased physical activity that usually occurs with age (Devlin 2000) places older people at greater risk of calcium deficiency, which accelerates the development of osteoporosis.

Arthritis

Arthritis, the main cause of disability in adults aged over 65 (Lueckenotte 2000), is a group of inflammatory or degenerative diseases that makes joints stiff, swollen and chronically painful. There are many (more than one hundred) types of arthritis; the two main types, osteoarthritis and rheumatoid arthritis, are discussed here.

Osteoarthritis is the most common form of chronic arthritis (Marieb 2001). Its progress is usually slow, but irreversible. Marieb (2001) suggests that years of compression and abrasion cause more cartilage to be destroyed than the body can replace. It is particularly prevalent in women, and most commonly occurs in the cervical and lumbar spine, and the fingers, knuckles, knees and hips (Marieb 2001).

The articular surfaces of cartilage become roughed and cracked, causing a typical crunching sound as they rub together. Anti-inflammatory drugs (e.g. aspirin, non-steroidal anti-inflammatories) can help relieve pain. Exercise helps maintain joint mobility, thus reducing osteoarthritis.

Rheumatoid arthritis is an autoimmune disease that is caused by massive infiltration of T lymphocytes and other cells into the synovial fluid of the joint (Ramsburg 2000). It usually begins after 40 years of age and affects women more than men (ratio 3:1) (Ramsburg 2000).

Rheumatoid arthritis can affect many joints, usually bilaterally. Typically, people with rheumatoid arthritis experience exacerbations and remissions, with progressive cartilage erosion and a formation of scar tissue. As scar tissue ossifies, bone ends fuse, immobilizing the joint (Marieb 2001). Rheumatoid arthritis causes chronic pain, but any loss of the ability to perform activities can also cause depression (Ramsburg 2000).

The chronic nature of rheumatoid arthritis creates many problems. In addition to medical treatments, the person should be encouraged to remain as active as possible, while allowing sufficient periods of rest between activity. Pain relief may be achieved through various complementary therapies, including use of heat and cold compresses, as well as through orthodox analgesics.

Teeth

Stereotypes of old age depict tooth loss. With good dental care, tooth loss can be reduced, but often not prevented. Fifty-seven per cent of 65–74-year-old and eighty per cent of people over 80 have no teeth (Devlin 2000). Many older people have partial or full dentures, and, owing to atrophy of the bones in the mouth, often experience problems with poorly fitting dentures (Schofield 1999).

Most tooth decay is caused by plaque, a film of sugar, bacteria and other debris that accumulates on teeth. Sugar, trapped between the tooth enamel and bacteria, is metabolized, producing metabolic acids, which destroy enamel. Plaque is especially likely to build up in crevices between the teeth and gums (the gingival crevice) (Mallett and Bailey 1996). Once it has accumulated, plaque calcifies to form a 'calculus' or 'tartar'. This calcification damages the seal between the gum (gingiva) and the teeth (Marieb 2001), causing gingivitis. With gingivitis, gums become sore and red, and bleed easily, especially when brushing teeth. Gingivitis can occur within a few days of plaque formation; so teeth should be kept clean, especially if people are not eating.

Plaque is not water soluble and so is difficult to remove. Brushing teeth regularly helps prevent accumulation, but will have little impact on any calcification. Any neglect of the teeth allows bacteria to invade and damage the bones that support the teeth (periodontitis/periodontal disease). Periodontitis affects up to 95% of people aged over 35, and causes 80–90% of adult tooth loss (Marieb 2001).

Tooth loss makes eating more difficult and so malnutrition more likely. The mouth is important for both verbal and non-verbal communication; smiling and kissing are likely to be considerably less attractive in someone with noticeable tooth loss. Therefore tooth loss can lead to social isolation.

Oral infections usually cause bad breath (halitosis), which is likely to cause further social isolation. They are also a source of possible infection elsewhere (e.g. respiratory, septicaemia). Therefore, in addition to the physical health, oral hygiene helps maintain social well-being. Immuno-compromised patients (e.g. those taking steroids) are especially at risk to opportunist infections, such as thrush (*Candida albicans*), a fungal infection that appears as a white coating in the mouth.

Oral hygiene in hospital is often less than ideal, partly because qualified nurses often lack sufficient knowledge about oral health (Adams 1996). A full oral assessment should be made of any clients at risk, including anyone unable to take an oral diet or to clean their teeth. Assessment requires a good light (e.g. a pen torch) and should identify:

- dental abnormalities
- plaque
- gingivitis
- colour of mucosa
- moisture/dryness.

Additional factors affecting oral health should be considered:

- disease
- inability or reluctance to eat
- drugs that will affect oral health (e.g. diuretics reduce salivary production).

Older people in institutions consume more sugar and so are most likely to suffer from tooth decay (Devlin 2000).

Oral hygiene should be maintained by cleaning the teeth with a toothbrush (small-headed toothbrushes are often easier for cleaning other people's teeth). The teeth should be brushed at least twice every day (Roberts 2000). If people find holding a toothbrush difficult, occupational therapists may be able to supply one with a special handle (Roberts 2000). Additional oral comfort may be provided by mouthwashes or moistened swabs/foam sticks. Admission to hospital may provide a useful opportunity for health promotion and advice or referral to specialist services. Calcified plaque is best removed by a dental hygienist. Other problems may benefit from referral to a dentist.

Dentures

Many older people wear partial or full dentures. Health assessment should identify whether patients normally wear them. Poorly fitting dentures, or failure to use them, contributes to malnutrition (Mojon et al 1999). Whenever possible, dentures should be worn as normal, to help eating and speaking and to support the normal shape of the mouth. If dentures are stored (including in patients' bedside lockers in hospitals), they should be stored safely, and a note kept of their location. On admission to hospital, dentures may be concealed in luggage; so staff should actively ask whether patients have dentures.

Dentures, like teeth, should be kept clean. They should be soaked in cold water (and any denture cleaning solutions the person normally uses). Water should be changed daily (Clarke 1993) to prevent infection. Ordinary toothpaste should not be used on dentures, as it can damage denture surfaces (Clarke 1993). Dentures may warp if soaked in hot water, or if left to dry (Clarke 1993). However, if dentures contain metal (sometimes found with partial dentures), water may cause corrosion; so they should not be soaked for more than 20 minutes (Jones 1998).

Conclusion

The integrity of the skin is fundamental to well-being. Understanding the principles of physiology and ageing is fundamental to prevention. This chapter has therefore explored some fundamental issues surrounding skincare. Specific pressure-area aids and wound-care dressings, which are well covered elsewhere, have not been discussed.

Reduction in muscle mass results in reduced strength. However, muscle loss is reduced by exercise; so the rate of muscle loss varies greatly between individuals. Muscular weakness affects many aspects of life; so people of all ages should be encouraged to use and build muscle tissue.

Age-related bone weakening is largely due to a loss of calcium stores. Osteoporosis, and resulting fractures, is more likely to occur when less calcium has been stored in adolescence and early adulthood. Many age-related pathologies of bone, such as arthritis, are often chronic and disabling.

The changes that occur to skin, bones and muscles affect many other systems in the body in a variety of ways. For example, reduced rib cage elasticity impairs breathing (Marieb 2001). Promoting and maintaining the health of skin, muscles and bones is therefore important for everyone. However, problems are more likely to occur in later life, making assessment and intervention by healthcare workers especially important.

References

Adams R (1996) Qualified nurses lack adequate knowledge related to oral health, resulting in inadequate oral care of patients on medical wards. Journal of Advanced Nursing 24 (3): 552–560.

Bowling A and Grant K (1992) Accidents in elderly care. Nursing Standard 6 (29): 28–30.

Cauley J A, Seeley D G, Ensrud K, Ettinger B, Black D, Cummings S R, Study of Osteoporotic Fracture Research Group (1995) Estrogen replacement therapy and fractures in older women. The study of osteoporotic fractures research group. Annals of Internal Medicine 122 (1): 9–16.

Clancy J and McVicar A (1995) Physiology and Anatomy. London: Edward Arnold.

Clarke G (1993) Mouthcare and the hospitalised patient. British Journal of Nursing 2 (4): 225–227.

Comstock G W, Burke A E, Hoffmann S C, Helzlsouer K J, Benduch A, Masi A T, Norkus E P, Malamet R L, Gershwin M E (1997) Serum concentrations of a tocopherol, B carotene, and retinol preceding the diagnosis of rheumatoid arthritis and systemic lupus erythematous. Annals of Rheumatic Diseases. 56 (5): 323–325.

Davies A J and Kenny R A (1996) Falls presenting to the Accident and Emergency Department: types of presentation and risk factor profile. Age and Ageing 25 (5): 362–366.

Dealey C (1992) Pressure sores, British Journal of Intensive Care, 2, 1, 34–39.

Devlin M (2000) The nutritional needs of the older person. Professional Nurse 16 (3): 951–955

Ganong W F (1999) Review of Medical Physiology 19th edn. Connecticut: Appleton & Lange.

Gray P and Hildebrand K (2000) Fall risk factors in Parkinson's disease. Journal of Neuroscience Nursing 32 (4): 222–228.

Herbert R A (1999) The biology of human ageing. In: Redfern S J and Ross F M (eds) Nursing Older People 3rd edn. pp. 55–77. Edinburgh: Churchill Livingstone.

Holt L (2000) Skeletal injuries. In: Dolan B and Holt L (eds) Accident & Emergency: theory into practice pp. 67–107. London: Baillière Tindall.

Hyatt R H, Whitelaw M N, Bhat A, Scott S, Maxwell J D (1990) Association of muscle strength with functional status of elderly people. Age and Ageing 19 (5): 330–336.

Jones C (1998) The importance of oral hygiene in nutritional support. British Journal of Nursing 7 (2): 74–83.

Koch T and Hudson S (2000) Older people and laxative abuse: literature review and pilot study report. Journal of Clinical Nursing 9 (4): 516–525.

Lowry M (1995) A pressure sore risk calculator in an Intensive Care unit. Intensive and Critical Care Nursing 9 (4): 226–231.

Lueckenotte AG (2000) Gerontologic Nursing 2nd edn. St Louis: Mosby.

Lufkin E G, Wahner H W, O'Fallon, Hodgson S F, Kotowicz M A, Lane A W, Judd H L, Caplan R H, Riggs B B (1992) Treatment of postmenopausal osteoporosis with transdermal oestrogen. Annals of Internal Medicine 117 (1): 1–9.

Mallett J and Bailey C (eds) (1996) The Royal Marsden NHS Trust Manual of Clinical Nursing Procedures 4th edn. Oxford: Blackwell Science.

Marieb EN (2001) Human Anatomy and Physiology 5th edn. San Francisco: Benjamin/Cummings Publishing Company Inc.

Mojon P, Budtz-Jorgensen E and Rapin C-H (1999) Relationship between oral health and nutrition in very old people. Age and Ageing 28 (5): 463–468.

Norton C (1996) The causes and nursing management of constipation. British Journal of Nursing 5 (20): 1252–1258.

Pellegrini V D and Evarts C M (1991) Systemic complications on injury. In: Rochwood C A, Green D P and Bucholz R W (eds) Fractures in adults volume 1 3rd edn. pp. 355–364. Philadelphia: J P Lippincott Company.

Quantock C and Benyon J (1994) Osteoporosis: condition of our time. Elderly Care 6 (6): 17–18.

Ramsburg K L (2000) Rheumatoid arthritis. American Journal of Nursing 100 (11): 40–44.

Reid J and Morison M (1994) Classification of pressure sore severity. Nursing Times 89 (42): 67–68.

Roberts J (2000) Developing an oral assessment and intervention tool for older people: 2. British Journal of Nursing 9 (18): 2033.

Sahota O and Masud T (1999) Osteoporosis: fact, fiction, fallacy and the future. Age and Ageing 28 (5): 425–428.

Schofield I (1999) Age-related changes. In: Heath H and Schofield I (eds) Healthy ageing: Nursing older people. pp. 81–101. London: Mosby.

Solomon E P, Schmidt R R and Adragna P (1990) Human Anatomy and Physiology 2nd edn. Fort Worth: Saunders College Publishing.

Tak P P and Bresnihan B (2000) The pathogenesis and prevention of joint damage in rheumatoid arthritis. Arthritis and Rheumatism 43 (12): 2619–2633.

Tingle J (1997) Pressure sores: counting the legal cost of nursing neglect. British Journal of Nursing 6 (13): 757–758.

Turner P A (2000) Osteoporosis – its causes and prevention: an update. Physiotherapy 16 (3): 135–149.

Waterlow J (1995) Pressure sores and their management. Care of the Critically Ill 11 (3): 121–125.

Wong D L, Huckleberry-Eaton M, Wilson D, Winkelstein M L, Ahmann E, DiVito-Thomas P (1999) Whaley & Wong's Nursing Care of Infants and Children 6th edn. St Louis: Mosby.

Wood S (2000) Osteoporosis. Geriatric Medicine 30 (9): 35–41.

CHAPTER 4

The cardiovascular system

PHILIP WOODROW

Introduction

The cardiovascular system comprises both the heart and the blood vessels. During a healthy life, degenerative changes occur in both parts of the system. Degenerative changes may be compounded by various pathophysiological processes. Some discussion of normal physiology is included in this chapter to help clarify how pathophysiology affects health.

The cardiovascular system is central to life, delivering oxygen and nutrients to nearly all body tissues. It is also a system that has historically been invested with major emotional connotations, as illustrated by amorous graffiti using images of the heart. So cardiovascular disease can be particularly threatening to the integrity of the person. This chapter focuses on the physiological changes that can occur in the cardiovascular system, rather than the emotional connotations compounding problems of the disease itself. However, health professionals planning patient care should be aware of the psychological issues involved.

Physiology

Except for capillaries, the cardiovascular system has three layers. In the blood vessels these are called the:

- tunica intima
- tunica media
- tunica adventitia.

In the heart the layers are called the:

- endocardium
- myocardium
- pericardium.

The functions of the respective layers are, however, essentially the same.

The tunica intima and the endocardium are smooth, thin layers of simple squamous epithelium. This provides a smooth surface to enable the easy flow of blood, and prevent thrombus formation. The tunica media and the myocardium are the muscle layers. Muscle controls the tone of tissue; so the more muscle present, the greater the ability to control the flow of blood and regulate its pressure. Different blood vessels have varying amounts of muscle. In the heart, the left ventricle, which pumps blood around the body, has more muscle than the right, which only pumps blood around the nearby lungs. In the vascular system, arterioles have most muscle, and veins least (see below). The tunica media and myocardium also have a collagen network, sometimes referred to as a 'skeleton' because they support the muscle-mass structure. The tunica adventitia and pericardium are the tough, fibrous outer layers that provide protection for the vessels and anchor them to the surrounding tissue.

The only blood vessels without three layers are the capillaries. Capillaries are made of single-layered epithelium. Having only a single layer enables fluids and solutes (nutrients, gases, waste products) to move into, and back from, the tissues. The sequence of blood vessels is normally arteries (leading from the heart) to arterioles, to capillaries, to venules, to veins (returning to the heart). Perfusion is essential to deliver and remove substances to and from the tissues. Ischaemia and impaired perfusion can affect almost any body tissue. An inadequate delivery of oxygen and nutrients, with an incomplete removal of waste, causes a loss of function, cell damage and, in some cases, a reduction in the size of organs.

Both the heart and blood vessels are controlled through a complex of higher (central nervous system) and local factors. Higher controls (from the cardiac and vasomotor centres in the hypothalamus) are transmitted through the sympathetic and parasympathetic nervous systems. With most body systems (except the gastrointestinal, where effects are reversed), the sympathetic system stimulates or increases, and the parasympathetic system relaxes or decreases. Most of the twelve cranial nerves are sympathetic; the main parasympathetic nerve is the vagus nerve (tenth cranial nerve), a nerve that has branches to all the main organs of the body.

Blood pressure

The cerebral regulation of blood pressure by the vasomotor centre relies on information from receptors, many of which are in the carotid sinuses (arteries to the brain), aortic arch and the walls of most large arteries in the neck and thorax. There are two types of receptors: *baroreceptors* and *chemoreceptors*. Baroreceptors respond to pressure, and chemoreceptors respond to chemicals (such as oxygen and acidity). While the function of chemoreceptors will decline with age, problems are more likely to occur because of a decline of baroreceptor function, which we shall now explore further.

When baroreceptors detect a reduction in blood pressure, they stimulate the arterioles to vasoconstrict. This increases systemic vascular resistance, which increases blood pressure. Chapter 2 describes the normal response to getting up from a supine position and how, with age, responses (mainly of the arterioles rather than the nervous system) are slower, causing a difference in blood pressure when lying and when standing, which increases the possibility of falls and fainting. Baroreceptors provide a homeostatic quick solution to a short-term problem, but can be 'reset' by chronic hypertension; this is a physiological response to protect the hypertensive person from inadequate perfusion, but can complicate chemical (drug) treatment of hypertension.

Blood pressure is the product of cardiac output (the amount of blood pumped out of the left ventricle every minute) and systemic vascular resistance (the resistance it meets in the body, primarily from the arterioles). This is usually expressed as the formula:

$$BP = CO \times SVR$$

Cardiac output is itself the product of stroke volume (the amount of blood ejected from the left ventricle with each contraction) and heart rate. So:

$$CO = SV \times HR$$

So the first formula can be rewritten:

$$BP = SV \times HR \times SVR$$

Blood pressure therefore depends on three factors:

- heart rate
- stroke volume
- systemic vascular resistance.

Changing one factor without altering the others will cause blood pressure to change correspondingly. However, homeostatic responses will normally try to compensate for any shortfall in one factor by increasing another. Therefore slower heart rates will either cause a fall in blood pressure or stimulate compensatory changes in either stroke volume or systemic vascular resistance.

Cardiac ageing

Various age-related changes occur in heart tissue. The atrioventricular node, part of the cardiac conduction system, thickens. This causes conduction to be delayed (prolonged PR interval on ECGs) between the atria and ventricles, which will reduce the heart rate.

Diseased hearts can develop many different (abnormal) rhythms, but atrial fibrillation, which causes an uncoordinated contraction of the atrial muscles, is the most common dysrhythmia (Lip and Beevers 1995). Atrial fibrillation is especially common in older people, occurring in 5% of over-65s in the UK and 10% of over-75s (Royal College of Physicians 1999). Atrial fibrillation increases myocardial oxygen consumption, while reducing cardiac output. If oxygen demand exceeds oxygen supply, heart muscle becomes ischaemic (angina – a sharp, stabbing pain in the chest) and, if not reversed, may infarct.

Atrial fibrillation may not be problematic enough to cause symptoms, in which case it would not normally be treated. But, if symptomatic, drugs (most often digoxin) will usually be prescribed to reduce the atrial rate. As well as reducing oxygen demand, the reduced atrial rate will enable the ventricles to fill more effectively and so increase the stroke volume (oxygen supply).

The heart and some veins (particularly the saphenous vein – the main vein in the legs) contain valves to prevent the backflow of blood. When a valve becomes stenotic, it becomes incompetent, allowing backflow. Cusps of heart valves thicken with age (Schofield 1999). Some diseases can also cause problems with heart valves. Rheumatic fever, a streptococcal infection, typically occurring around puberty, stimulates the production of antibodies to the streptococcus that may cross-react with the body's own proteins (Abbas et al 1994), causing stenosis of heart valves in later life. The mitral valve, between the right atrium and ventricle, is most often affected. Although rheumatic fever can now be easily treated with penicillin, some older people caught rheumatic fever before the widespread availability of penicillin. In the future, the numbers of older people with valve disease caused by rheumatic fever should decline. But twentieth-century improvements in cardiac surgery have increased the survival of people with congenital defects. As these generations grow older, the number of people with valve disease due to congenital defects is increasing in industrialized countries.

In the heart, backflow increases the workload of and the demand for myocardial oxygen, while reducing output and myocardial oxygen supply. If myocardial oxygen demand exceeds supply, muscle becomes ischaemic. Severe heart valve disease may necessitate surgical replacement of the valves. Hardening of valves in the main veins of the legs causes varicose veins. Varicose veins result in pooling of blood within these veins, causing oedema and a reduction in the amount of blood returned to the heart. Varicose veins can be 'stripped', an operation involving the removal of valves and therefore the widening of the lumen of the blood vessel, but without replacing the valves which would help prevent backflow.

Vascular ageing

With age, collagen fibres cross-link and the amount of smooth muscle in the arterial walls increases (Herbert 1999, Schofield 1999). The cross-linking of collagen, together with calcium deposits, increases vascular resistance, thus reducing the ability of the blood vessels to dilate, a significant factor in the development of hypertension. Systemic vascular resistance increases by about 1 per cent every year from the age of 40 (Herbert 1999). With age, capillary endothelium thickens, reducing the permeability of their walls (Herbert 1999), and thus reducing tissue perfusion. Calcium deposits in the blood vessel walls make the muscle bone-like, and thus less flexible. In the myocardium, ventricular filling is limited by reduced muscle stretch, thus reducing stroke volume.

Although ageing is inevitable, most cardiovascular systems are robust enough to withstand many insults. A healthy lifestyle (including exercise) can delay cardiovascular ageing symptoms such as hypertension (Kasch et al 1999).

Atherosclerosis

Most cardiovascular disease is an accumulation of years of insults to the system. Some of these insults are inflicted by lifestyle (e.g. diet and smoking), others by the normal ageing process (e.g. collagen deposits). The result of continued damage to the blood vessels is atherosclerosis: a hardening of the blood vessels. Atherosclerosis causes, or significantly contributes to:

- thrombus formation (e.g. deep-vein thrombosis)
- hypertension
- ischaemia
- emboli.

Atherosclerosis is the accumulation of:

- lipid
- collagen
- calcium deposits

in the normally smooth inner walls of arteries (tunica intima) (Woolf 2000).

This accumulation builds a fibrous, hard cap that facilitates platelet deposition, and so thrombus formation, within the lumen of the artery (Todd 1997). If part of the thrombus breaks off, an embolus travels through the cardiovascular system until it reaches a blood vessel that is too small for it to pass through. The capillaries beyond the blockage will not be perfused, and so will infarct. Infarction may occur in any tissue, but is most likely to cause problems in the brain (cerebrovascular accident – CVA), heart (myocardial infarction) and lungs (pulmonary embolus).

Blood vessels produce various homeostatic chemicals, such as nitric oxide, which influence the dilation of muscle walls, and so lumen size. So, for example, hypoxia stimulates endothelium to release nitric oxide. Nitric oxide relaxes arterial muscle, thus increasing blood flow into the ischaemic tissue. The stimulus for nitric oxide production is removed once the ischaemia is resolved. However, nitric oxide is produced only by intact endothelium and so will not be produced in atherosclerosed vessels (Todd 1997). So, at the same time that the blood flow is reduced by a narrowing of the lumen, the body loses its ability to autoregulate. The hypoxic myocardium is thus at greater risk of infarction. For example, people with symptoms of coronary heart disease (CHD) (discussed below) have severe atherosclerosis and so lack the ability to significantly increase myocardial blood supply to meet any increase in myocardial oxygen demand. This limits their ability to increase most physical activities.

Although there is some genetic predisposition to atherosclerosis, there are many other factors that influence it. Oestrogen provides significant protection against atherosclerosis; so rates are generally significantly lower in pre-menopausal women than in men of the same age. This explains the ten- to fifteen-year gap between rates of myocardial infarctions among men and women under about 50 years of age (Solomon et al 1990). However, the sudden fall in oestrogen levels during and following menopause rapidly accelerates atherosclerosis formation in women (Walling et al 1988).

High blood cholesterol significantly contributes to atherosclerosis. Cholesterol is a chemical occurring naturally in the body, and some cholesterol is necessary for healthy body function. However, many people have excessive levels in their blood. Cholesterol is widely found in saturated fats (mainly animal fats). In contrast, some mono- and polyunsaturated fats can reduce blood cholesterol. For example, prolonged intake (two years of 1.5 g/day) of omega 3 polyunsaturated fatty acids (found in fish oils) can reduce atherosclerosis (von Schacky et al 1999). Omega 6 polyunsaturated fatty acids (e.g. sunflower, soya bean oil) can also reduce cholesterol levels (Wasling 1999).

Atherosclerosis reduces the blood flow to the tissues. This causes various problems with other systems that are particularly associated with the latter years of life. For example, cerebral blood flow reduces by 20% (Herbert 1999), leading to possible transient ischaemic attacks (TIAs), cerebrovascular accidents (CVAs), confusion and (organic) dementia. Effects on some other systems will be covered in the next chapter.

Coronary heart disease

Even at rest, heart muscle extracts 70–80% of available oxygen (Ganong 1999); so a healthy heart has relatively little physiological reserve between the onset of symptoms of hypoxia and ischaemic tissue death. Reduced respiratory function and cardiovascular ageing further decrease functional reserve.

Cardiovascular disease is usually the accumulation of factors over a lifetime; by the age of 12–15 most people in the UK have the signs of coronary artery disease, but symptoms usually occur only when there is a 70% occlusion. So hypertension remains asymptomatic for many years (Marieb, 2001, suggests 10–20 years), causing progressive strain on the cardiovascular system. As the heart is forced to pump against ever-increasing resistance, the muscle around the left ventricle enlarges (hypertrophies), a compensatory mechanism to meet increased demand. But the larger muscle mass inevitably becomes less elastic and so less able to respond to fluctuations in demand. A larger muscle mass also consumes more oxygen. If cardiac output fails to supply sufficient oxygen to the cardiac muscle itself, the myocardium becomes ischaemic.

Microcirculation (the capillary system) is dynamic, responding to demands from the body. Therefore, if flow through one capillary is blocked, another capillary usually develops to bypass the problem. These bypass capillaries are called 'collateral circulation'. Collateral vessels are typically small, weak and tortuous but can provide sufficient flow to relieve symptoms of myocardial ischaemia (angina). Therefore, although the incidence of myocardial infarction in the under-50s is significantly higher in men than in women, men surviving to 50 years of age have usually developed a considerable collateral circulation system. When post-menopausal women are suddenly exposed to the ravages of coronary arteriosclerosis, they lack a significant protective collateral circulatory system. A lack of collateral circulation causes post-menopausal women to suffer more severe cardiac disease and have a higher mortality than men of the same age. The use of hormone replacement therapy does not appear to reduce the incidence of atherosclerosis in post-menopausal women (Herrington et al 2000).

Various drugs, especially nitrates (e.g. GTN), may relieve angina. But the risk of myocardial infarction and the impaired quality of life may necessitate cardiac surgery. However, some people are too frail to undergo cardiac surgery and therefore have to live with this disabling and potentially fatal disease.

Hypertension

Hypertension is a frequent problem among older people. The World Health Organisation defines hypertension as a sustained arterial blood pressure greater than 160/95 (Wingard et al 1991); Marieb (2001) suggests that 30% of people over 50 are hypertensive, a figure probably applicable to the UK.

Hypertension can be classified as either primary or secondary. Secondary hypertension is where some other physiological or pathological process is causing hypertension (such as certain endocrine disorders). With secondary hypertension, the underlying cause should be treated. However, 90% of hypertension is primary (Marieb 2001), where there is no triggering disease process causing the hypertension, although various factors will have provoked the problem. Due to its insidious, but progressive, nature, hypertension is often called a 'silent killer' (Marieb 2001). Various factors have been detected in hypertension. Some, such as stress, 'Type A' personality and heredity, are difficult to change. Other factors are more amenable to change; of these, smoking and diet/obesity are discussed below.

Systemic vascular disease

The supply of oxygen and nutrients to tissues, and the removal of waste products, relies on perfusion. Perfusion occurs at a capillary level. As capillaries are the smallest blood vessels, they are most likely to be affected by poor perfusion.

Hypoxic metabolism stimulates pain receptors (nociceptors), causing cramp. Cramps are experienced by anyone exercising significantly beyond the limits their bodies are used to. But cramp can occur in any ischaemic tissue. Just as ischaemic heart muscle can cause angina, so people with ischaemic skeletal muscle often experience cramp pain, especially overnight when blood becomes more viscous, thus reducing blood flow. Half of people over 70 years of age have peripheral vascular disease (Lueckenotte 2000).

Sudden cramp may be relieved by rubbing the skin above the affected area, which stimulates blood flow. Persistent cramp should be medically investigated. Many people suffering from night cramps benefit from quinine.

Smoking

Smoking has many harmful effects on the body, most of which have been recognized for many years. Nevertheless, the incidence of smoking remains high. While staff should not blame people who have diseases caused by smoking, reducing or stopping smoking will reduce or prevent future problems, regardless of the person's age or existing problems (Herbert 1999). Therefore, healthcare should have a positive role in promoting health through encouraging people (and their relatives) to reduce or stop smoking. So awareness of the effects of smoking is important for both health professionals and patients. Smoking exposes the body to many harmful substances, especially:

- nicotine
- tar
- carbon monoxide.

Nicotine is a powerful stimulant of the sympathetic nervous system – an intravenous injection of the nicotine from one packet of cigarettes into a non-smoker would probably be fatal. As identified earlier:

$$BP = SV \times HR \times SVR$$

Nicotine increases the heart rate and systemic vascular resistance, and increases circulating cholesterol levels; so smoking contributes (significantly) to atherosclerosis, hypertension and coronary artery disease (Scrutton 1992). Nicotine is more addictive than heroin (Haas and Hass 1990), yet remains a socially accepted and legal drug. As tolerance to nicotine develops, the body is able to tolerate larger and larger doses. Although smoking uptake peaked in people born between 1910 and 1920 (Connolly 1996), and there are some legal restrictions on tobacco advertising and sales in the UK, numbers of smokers among all adult and teenage cohorts remain a cause for concern.

The tar in cigarettes is the same as any other tar. Remembering what a newly tarred footpath does to shoes gives a good impression of what tar does to human (and experimental animal) lungs. Human airways are lined with a coating of fine hairs called cilia, which waft mucous and foreign bodies (such as bacteria) up the airway so they can either be swallowed and removed from the body through the gut or coughed out. As tar on roads holds loose chippings together, so tar in human airways holds the cilia together, preventing them from functioning. Thus debris and foreign organisms accumulate in the lungs, predisposing smokers to hypoxia and chest infections. About 70% of the tar in cigarette smoke is deposited in the lungs (O'Connell 2000).

A relatively short break from smoking enables cilia to regain some function. So, after a night's sleep without smoking, cilia make some recovery. The return of cilial function stimulates a cough reflex, an attempt to remove foreign materials (such as tar) from the respiratory tract. This early-morning cough usually troubles smokers, who too often resume smoking to stop the cough. The cigarette stops the cough by re-disabling cilia. So what smokers consider a 'cure' only makes the real problem worse, as well as adding to circulating nicotine levels.

Smoke contains more than 4000 compounds, many of which are toxic (Health Education Authority 1997). Probably the main toxin is carbon monoxide, although cigarette smoke also contains many free radicals (Heunks and Dekhuijzen 2000). Carbon monoxide is a tasteless, odourless and invisible poison. It has more than 200 times the affinity for haemoglobin that oxygen has (Harvey and Hutton 1999) and so prevents oxygen being carried by the blood. Severe carbon monoxide poisoning causes about one thousand deaths each year in the UK (Harvey and Hutton 1999).

Small amounts of carbon monoxide are normally produced in the body, but, whereas non-smokers normally have blood levels of about 2%, smokers have 3%–8% (Hawkins et al 2000), rising to about 10% with heavy smokers and about 20% with cigar smokers (Harvey and Hutton 1999). Although far less than the often-fatal levels found in fire victims, this causes generalized tissue hypoxia, which over many years of smoking will accelerate cell dysfunction and damage.

Smoking has many other harmful effects; so anyone pretending that smoking is harmless is living under a very dangerous delusion. Some smokers will be lucky enough not to harm their bodies enough through smoking to trigger diseases or cause significant problem. But who the lucky smokers will be remains unpredictable. Unfortunately, smokers too often resort to denial: their father/mother/uncle/aunt smoked all their life and lived to a ripe old age.

Some damage cannot be reversed, but other parts of the human body show remarkable abilities to repair and recover (e.g. cilia). At the very least, stopping smoking prevents any further harm.

In addition to harm caused to themselves, passive smoking harms others around them. Young children are particularly susceptible to the effects of passive smoking (Gidding and Schydlower 1994). Prohibiting smoking in hospital protects the rights and health of other non-smoking patients, staff and visitors. But healthcare staff should be careful about dictating choices to patients. Instead, information should be made available to help patients make informed choices about their own lifestyle.

Diet and obesity

These two factors are often, although not always, linked together. Denial of the problem of overeating too often leads to excuses of 'heredity' obesity. Heredity obesity occurs in only about 5% of the population (Marieb 2001). Obesity is usually caused by eating too much, or the wrong type of, food, often compounded by using too little energy. Fat provides energy stores for the body, but each excess 9.3 calories is stored as one gram of fat (Guyton and Hall 2000). However, few people in affluent societies need to draw significantly on fat energy stores, therefore persistent excess of energy intake over energy expenditure results in obesity. Basal metabolic rate falls with age. Devlin (2000) suggests that the basal metabolic rate of a 70-year-old is 9–12% less than it was at 25 years of age (Devlin 2000). So, less energy is consumed. If energy intake remains unchanged, unused energy fuels will be stored as fat. However, many older people experience reduced appetite.

Obesity is calculated by body mass index (BMI): the person's weight in kilograms divided by the square of their height in metres. To help staff calculate body mass index, and identify whether the person is under-weight (<20), ideal (20–25), overweight (25–30), or obese (>30) (DOH 1994), charts are widely available. Charts should be gender specific, as figures will be slightly higher in women (Sanders and Bazalgette, 1994, recommend an ideal female BMI of 26-28).

There are close links between health and body mass index. Mortality rates are lowest among men with BMI of 23.5–24.9 and women with a BMI of 22.0–23.4 (Calle et al 1999), increasing sharply when BMI exceeds 30 (Adams and Murphy 2000). Ill health significantly increases when BMI exceeds 25 (Gibbs 1996), with premature deaths doubling in people with a BMI of over 35 (Adams and Murphy 2000). This ill health places increased demand upon health services. *The Health of the Nation* (DOH 1992) set targets to reduce obesity among men aged 16-64 from 8% to 6% and among women of the same age from 12% to 8%. Perhaps people above retirement age were excluded from these targets on the (stereotypic) assumption that they are not economically productive. However, obesity is an increasing problem among older people and one area where staff can develop useful health promotion initiatives.

Stereotypes of older people living off bread, butter, jam, tea and biscuits are unsubstantiated (Tinker 1997). However, lifestyles may predispose them to extremes of either malnourishment or obesity. More older people are obese than underweight. Devlin (2000) finds that 60% of people in the community and 40% of people in institutions have a BMI of below 25. People are more likely to be underweight in institutions than in the community (Devlin 2000). Social factors, such as a lack of exercise and finance, will accentuate these trends. As an affluent generation retires, increasing numbers of the 'young old' live a comfortable lifestyle that can support overeating and obesity (together with an overuse of cars, which reduces exercise further). Saturated (animal) fats are especially likely to cause obesity (Marieb 2001), as well as raising blood cholesterol. Older people eat excessive saturated fats (Devlin 2000).

Systemic vascular resistance is affected by the length of the blood vessel. Just as a light dimmer switch works by increasing or decreasing the length of wire through which a current passes, so increasing unnecessary body tissue (fat) increases the total length of the cardiovascular system.

Increased length means increased resistance and so raised blood pressure. Obesity is a major factor in hypertension, heart disease, myocardial infarction, arteriosclerosis, and diabetes mellitus (and other disease processes).

There has recently been much media speculation about the beneficial effects of alcohol to the cardiovascular system. The currently limited and controversial knowledge base allows the provisional conclusion that moderate intakes of some alcohols may be beneficial. Unfortunately, media hype is too often used as an excuse for excess. Stereotypes of the 'social drinker' being a heavy drinker have a large element of truth; the extent of alcoholism in old age is often underestimated (Scrutton 1992). Excess of any substance is likely to be harmful, and alcohol is no exception. Alcohol (particularly beer) is high in carbohydrates. So alcohol provides energy source (although lacking the proteins also necessary for health), which, like other energy sources, can lead to obesity (e.g. 'beer bellies') and hypertension.

Conclusion

Normal ageing occurs in all parts of the cardiovascular system, and, as the cardiovascular system is the transport system for most of the body, symptoms of cardiovascular disease can affect any other system. There is little that can be done to delay or prevent normal ageing. But the effects of normal ageing are compounded by a variety of added insults from chosen lifestyles. Staff can inform people how to minimize or at least reduce harmful factors, enabling people to make an informed choice about their future lifestyle.

Cardiovascular health affects all other systems of the body; many problems identified here will be discussed further in the next chapter, which gives an overview of how other body systems can be affected by the ageing process.

References

Abbas A K, Lichtman A H and Pober J S (1994) Cellular and Molecular Immunology 2nd edn. Philadelphia: W B Saunders.

Adams J P and Murphy P G (2000) Obesity of anaesthesia and intensive care. British Journal of Anaesthesia 85 (1): 91–108.

Calle E E, Thun M J, Petrelli J M, Rodriguez C, Heath C W (1999) Body-mass index and mortality in a prospective cohort of U.S. adults. New England Journal of Medicine 341 (15): 1097–1105.

Connolly M J (1996) Obstructive airways disease: a hidden disability in the aged. Age and Ageing 25 (4): 265–267.

Department of Health (1992) The Health of the Nation. London: HMSO.

Department of Health (1994) Nutritional aspects of cardiovascular disease. Committee on medical aspects of food policy. Report on health and social subjects 46. London: HMSO.

Devlin M (2000) The nutritional needs of the older person. Professional Nurse 16 (3): 951–955.

Ganong W F (1999) Review of Medical Physiology 19th edn. Connecticut: Appleton & Lange.

Gibbs W W (1996) Gaining on fat. Scientific American 274 (8): 70–76.

Gidding S and Schydlower M (1994) Active and passive tobacco exposure. Pediatrics 94: 750–1.

Guyton A C and Hall J E (2000) Textbook of Medical Physiology 10th edn. Philadelphia: W B Saunders Company.

Haas F and Hass S (1990) The chronic bronchitis and emphysema handbook. Chichester: John Wiley and Sons.

Harvey W R and Hutton P (1999) Carbon monoxide: chemistry, role, toxicity and treatment. Current Anaesthesia and Critical Care 10 (3): 158–163.

Hawkins M, Harrison J and Charters P (2000) Severe carbon monoxide poisoning: outcome after hyperbaric oxygen therapy. British Journal of Anaesthesia 84 (5): 584–586.

Health Education Authority (1997) National smoking education campaign. Fact Sheets. London: HEA.

Herbert R A (1999) The biology of human Ageing. In: Redfern S J and Ross F M (eds) Nursing Older People 3rd edn. pp. 55–77. Edinburgh: Churchill Livingstone.

Herrington D M, Reboussin D M, Brosnihan K B, Sharp P C, Shumaker S A, Snyder T E, Furberg C D, Kowalchuk G J, Stuckey T D, Rogers W J, Givens D H, Waters D (2000) Effects of estrogen replacement on the progression of coronary-artery atherosclerosis. New England Journal of Medicine 343 (6): 522–529.

Heunks L M A and Dekhuijzen P N R (2000) Respiratory muscle function and free radicals: from cell to COPD. Thorax 55 (8): 704–716.

Kasch F W, Boyer J L, Schmidt P K, Wells R H, Wallace J P, Verity L S, Guy H, Schneider D (1999) Ageing of the cardiovascular system during 33 years of aerobic exercise. Age and Ageing 28 (6): 531–536.

Lip G Y H and Beevers D G (1995) History, epidemiology and importance of atrial fibrillation. British Medical Journal 311 (7016): 1361–1363.

Lueckenotte AG (2000) Gerontologic Nursing 2nd edn. St Louis: Mosby.

Marieb E N (2001) Human Anatomy and Physiology 5th edn. San Francisco: Benjamin/Cummings Publishing Company Inc.

O'Connell L (2000) Management of patients with chronic obstructive pulmonary disease in ICU and promotion of smoking cessation. Nursing in Critical Care 5 (3): 130–136.

Royal College of Physicians (1999) Atrial fibrillation in hospital and general practice: a consensus statement. British Journal of Cardiology 6 (3): 138–140.

Sanders T and Bazalgette P (1994) You Don't Have To Diet. London: Bantam Press.

Schofield I (1999) Age-related changes. In: Heath H and Schofield I (eds) Healthy Ageing: Nursing Older People pp. 81–101. London: Mosby.

Scrutton S (1992) Ageing, Healthy and in Control. London: Chapman & Hall.

Solomon E P, Schmidt R R and Adragna P J (1990) Human Anatomy and Physiology 2nd edn. Fort Worth: Saunders College Publishing.

Tinker A (1997) Older People in Modern Society 4th edn. London: Longman.

Todd N (1997) The physiological knowledge required by nurses working in caring for patients with unstable angina. Nursing in Critical Care 2 (1): 17–24.

von Schacky C, Angerer P, Kothny W, Theisen K, Mudra H (1999) The effect of dietary omega-3 fatty acids on coronary atherosclerosis. A randomised, double-blind, placebo-controlled trial. Annals of Internal Medicine 130 (7): 554–562.

Walling A, Tremblay G J L, Jobin J, Charest J, Delage F, Leblanc M H, Tessier Y, Villa J (1988) Evaluating the rehabilitation potential of a large population of post-myocardial infarction patients: adverse prognosis for women. Journal of Cardiopulmonary Rehabilitation 8: 99–106.

Wasling C (1999) Role of the cardioprotective diet in preventing coronary heart disease. British Journal of Nursing 8 (18): 1239–1248.

Wingard L B, Brody T M, Larner J and Schwartz A (1991) Human Pharmacology: molecular to clinical. London: Wolfe Publishing Limited.

Woolf N (2000) Cell, Tissue and Disease 3rd edn. Edinburgh: W B Saunders Company Ltd.

CHAPTER 5

Further aspects of physiological ageing

PHILIP WOODROW

Introduction

Previous chapters have explored how ageing affects a single system. This chapter provides an overview of how ageing can affect the respiratory, gastrointestinal, central nervous and genitourinary systems. This overview supplements the breadth of understanding needed to plan holistic care. Some more-frequently encountered disease processes and problems affecting older people are introduced, with special focus on:

- diabetes mellitus
- constipation
- Parkinson's disease
- CVAs.

However, in developing breadth, this chapter inevitably cannot provide the depth that professionals working in specialist areas may need.

Dividing this section of the book by body systems has enabled each to be focused on individually. However, each person functions as a whole and not as a collection of independent systems. Inevitably, this chapter overlaps with material elsewhere. Dental health affects nutrition, which was discussed in Chapter 3, while obesity was discussed in Chapter 4. Discussion focuses on organic pathologies, such as Parkinson's disease, rather than on psychological health. However, physiology and psychology are parts of the whole person; so, whatever medical diagnosis is made, each person should be approached holistically, their care meeting both physiological and psychological needs.

The respiratory system

Traditional divisions between the respiratory and cardiovascular systems are physiologically largely artificial. Both are essential to carry oxygen from the atmosphere into the cells, and to remove carbon dioxide (a waste product of cell metabolism) from the cells. Alveolar and tissue-gas exchange both require adequate perfusion. But pulmonary circulation is affected by similar ageing and pathological processes to systemic circulation; so, with age, pulmonary perfusion reduces, making gas diffusion less effective.

Changes to lung tissue occur as part of 'normal' ageing. It becomes less elastic (Herbert 1999), which increases the rate of work necessary to maintain adequate breathing (the amount of oxygen consumed by respiratory muscles), and thus reduces the proportion of oxygen available for other tissues. Respiratory muscles, like other muscles, become weaker with age and so become less able to compensate. A 90-year-old has, on average, half the pulmonary function of a 30-year-old (Hough 1996). Reduced reserve function makes many older people prone to shortness of breath, respiratory infection and other diseases.

All the upper airway, and part of the lower airway, is lined with cilia: tiny hairs that filter inhaled air. Cilia prevent dust and other particles larger than 10 micrometres (Rhoades and Pflanzer 1996) from reaching the alveoli, and waft mucus upwards so that it can either be swallowed or coughed out. With age, the number and effectiveness of cilia are reduced (Herbert 1999), increasing the likelihood of chest infection.

Other respiratory-tract changes result from exposure to toxic substances, although vary greatly between individuals. Factors affecting development of chronic respiratory disease include:

- smoking
- where people have lived
- lifestyle
- occupational exposure (e.g. silicosis, asbestosis)
- individual response to toxins.

Susceptibility varies over the course of each lifespan, tissue being most susceptible to damage during childhood.

Smoking, a major cause of airway disease, was discussed in Chapter 4. Combined effects of normal ageing and toxic damage on the respiratory system can result in chronic respiratory insufficiency. Older people often suffer from a range of chronic illnesses, some of which may be severely disabling. Renwick and Connolly (1995) found that 30% of people aged over 45 suffered from asthma or bronchitis. Although higher than previously reported figures, the authors acknowledge that the study being undertaken in Manchester may have affected results. However, chronic obstructive pulmonary disease in older people is more common than diagnosis rates would suggest (Connolly 1996).

Acute infections can also cause problems, ranging from breathlessness to respiratory failure. Older people are more likely to catch acute infections due to a reduced function of the immune system and increased risk factors (e.g. reduced mobility). Acute infections will exacerbate any underlying chronic condition. When lying down (especially if feeding or being fed lying down), people are also at risk of aspirating stomach contents, which can cause aspiration pneumonia. Staff planning and providing care should therefore consider all existing and potential problems.

Breathlessness, an early sign of tissue hypoxia, is distressing. As the body is starved of oxygen, the person will display a range of symptoms, ranging from fear and aggression to lethargy and tiredness. Activities such as feeding and sleeping become difficult when breathless; so the energy supply is likely to be reduced, while oxygen consumption is increased. Many breathless people find high-calorie drinks easier to manage than solid meals. If oxygen therapy is needed, nasal cannulae leave the mouth free for eating, drinking and talking. However, nasal cannulae are unsuitable for more than 6 litres of oxygen per minute (Hough 1996); so only relatively low percentages of oxygen can be delivered (precise percentages depend on breath size).

When planning care, staff should assess each person's functional ability and limitations, offering help and advice to achieve their maximum potential. Respiratory disease is often disabling, and, although full recovery is not always possible, health advice can improve quality of life.

The gastrointestinal system

The gut both absorbs nutrition and removes waste. Both functions can cause significant problems.

Adequate nutrition for older people can be problematic. Obesity is discussed in Chapter 4. Malnutrition can include low intake (quantity) but, in Western societies, is more often caused by an inadequate supply of nutrients to meet metabolic demands (quality). So someone eating mainly bread or biscuits may maintain a sufficient quantity, but not quality, of intake. Reasons for malnutrition may be economic, psychological or physiological. Economic factors, such as poverty, and psychological factors, such as a lack of motivation to cook for one, are not developed here. Dental decay and gum recession (see Chapter 3) increase eating difficulties, while reduced numbers of taste-sense receptors make food less appetizing (Eliopoulos 1997). Devlin (2000) found that 84% of patients in one long-stay hospital had calorie intakes below their esti-mated energy expenditure. While this may be an isolated extreme, and was not reflected by patients in the community, it is a cause for concern.

Salivary production is stimulated through a reflex response to food (and other objects) in the mouth. Saliva lubricates and cleans the mouth. Although mainly composed of water, it also contains small, but import-ant, amounts of various chemicals, including various antibacterial substances (immunoglobulin A, lysozyme and lactoferrin) and proline-rich proteins (which protect tooth enamel). Reduced salivary secretion therefore increases the risk of oral infection, mouth ulcers and tooth decay.

Salivary production decreases with age; so older people are more likely to develop problems. Someone unable to eat usually produces less saliva; what is produced will be tenacious, warm and largely static, and so forms a medium for bacterial growth. Reduced blood flow to the salivary glands (e.g. from shock or diuretic drugs) will reduce salivary production. Oral assessment should identify risk factors so that additional mouth-washes and other care can be provided as needed.

People being treated with diuretics, and who have incontinence or limited mobility, may attempt to reduce their needs to urinate by reduc-ing their fluid intake. This apparently logical reasoning, however, is likely to increase gut-water absorption, thus causing constipation (see below). Urinary stasis also increases the risk of urinary-tract infection. Normal fluid-intake volumes should therefore be encouraged.

Most nutrients are absorbed in the small intestine. Villi, finger-like projections from the bowel wall into the lumen, increase surface area for nutrient absorption. With age, villi become shorter and broader, thus reducing absorption (Herbert 1999). However, age-related, reduced-basal energy demands together with reserve function may prevent reduced gut absorption being problematic for the person.

Water is the main nutrient absorbed in the colon, and so age-related atrophy of mucosal and muscular layers in the large intestine make older people prone to dehydration. Reduced muscle mass also reduces peristal-sis. Both of these, and many other factors, can cause constipation.

Even when adequate nutrients are absorbed, reduced pancreatic func-tion may cause inadequate circulating levels of insulin. Insulin transports blood glucose across cell walls, providing energy for all cells in the body. So, when there are inadequate levels of insulin to supply body needs (diabetes mellitus – see below), inappropriately high blood-glucose levels are created, while cells are starved of their energy source.

The liver has a complex series of functions. Among its gastrointestinal functions are detoxification and storage (of glucose and trace elements, such as iron and vitamins). Between early adulthood and late old age liver mass decreases by about one-third (Storer 1996). This reduces the capacity to store nutrients (Herbert 1999), and removal of toxins from the body becomes less efficient (Rebenson-Piano 1989). Toxicity may cause confusion (Schwertz and Buschmann 1989). Slower detoxification is the reason why older people often need smaller dosages of therapeutic drugs than would be given to younger people. However, multiple pathology often creates a need for polypharmacy, causing possible interactions and further toxicity. People and their carers should be aware of the possible adverse effects of drugs. Before labelling someone as confused, the possible effects of drugs should be considered.

Diabetes mellitus

Diabetes insipidus and diabetes mellitus (more often just called 'diabetes') are two totally different and unrelated pathologies, and, despite their shared name, should not be confused. Diabetes insipidus is a disorder of the pituitary gland, resulting in an insufficient production of antidiuretic hormone; it is not discussed further in this book. Diabetes mellitus, insulin dysfunction, is usually caused by a lack of production in the pancreas. When the word 'diabetes' is used without any suffix, it almost invariably refers to diabetes mellitus. This convention is followed in this text.

About 2% of people in the UK (Marshall 1996) suffer from diabetes mellitus. There are two types of diabetes mellitus, classified by the World Health Organisation (1980) as types 1 and 2. Other (older) names, such as 'juvenile', 'early-onset' or 'insulin-dependent' for type 1, and 'late-onset' and 'non-insulin-dependent' for type 2, should no longer be used, but sometimes still are; so readers should be able to recognize their meaning.

Type 1 diabetes tends to begin early in life, especially between 11 and 12 years of age (Abbas et al 1994). Extensive destruction of the beta cells (which produce insulin) in the pancreas (Abbas et al 1994), often with additional insulin antagonism within the bloodstream, results in a severe lack of insulin. Type 1 diabetes may be due to various causes, especially autoimmune disorders (Abbas et al 1994). Regular insulin supplements will be needed with type 1 diabetes.

Type 2 is caused by age-related atrophy of the pancreas, usually occurring after the age of 40 (Dunning and Martin 1998). This is slowly progressive, but rarely (except in very late stages) as severe as type 1 diabetes and so can often be controlled by diet. Some people with type 2 diabetes also need regular oral hypoglycaemic medication. Most (85%) diabetics have type 2 diabetes (Dunning and Martin 1998). A partial pancreatectomy (e.g. for secondary carcinoma) inevitably reduces insulin production and so will probably cause diabetes.

Both types of diabetes mellitus share this feature of insufficient insulin. Insulin is used to transport glucose and other sugars from the blood into the cells, where the sugars are needed for energy production. Insulin normally keeps blood sugar levels between 4 and 8 mmol per litre; so insufficient insulin causes hyperglycaemia. Insulin insufficiency may be caused by a lack of production or by antagonists to insulin function.

Pancreatic function may be impaired by drugs that antagonize the effects of insulin (for example, some antihypertensive agents). With drug-induced diabetes, the body may produce as much insulin as before, but antagonists cause a need for more insulin. Drug-induced diabetes can be 'cured' by stopping the insulin antagonist (although dangers of removing the offending drug should be considered; so this should be done under medical or pharmaceutical supervision). The hormone cortisol, released in response to stress, is an insulin antagonist. Therefore people experiencing severe stress (e.g. illness, surgery) who have limited pancreatic reserve may develop hyperglycaemia. Removing the stressor should therefore restore the patient's ability to maintain normal blood-sugar levels, although drug- or stress-induced diabetes suggests the person has limited reserve function and so is at risk of developing type 2 diabetes.

Prolonged hyperglycaemia can cause various complications:

• atherosclerosis
• coronary heart disease and myocardial infarction
• chronic renal failure
• nerve damage
• blindness.

People with diabetes are at significantly greater risk of developing disease; so their diabetes should be controlled to maintain blood sugar at a high enough level to provide glucose for cell metabolism, without being excessively high. A general rule of thumb for managing diabetes is therefore to maintain blood-sugar levels at just slightly higher than normal (aim for 10 mmol per litre), or just high enough to cause a trace of glycosuria.

Many foods contain sugars. Simple sugars, which are absorbed directly into the bloodstream, should be avoided as far as possible in diabetes. Carbohydrates are also converted into blood sugar within the body, but this process takes longer; so fluctuations in blood sugar between meals are less uneven. Increasing dietary fibre also delays absorption of carbohydrate-derived sugars and so improves the control of blood sugar.

Without adequate glucose, mitochondria within cells use other fuels (fats and body proteins) for metabolism. The use of body fat and protein causes tissue wasting, and also produces significantly more metabolic waste products (such as lactic acid and ketones). Ketones are easily detected both in blood and urine. The process of burning body fat for fuel is called *ketosis*. Normal blood-ketone levels are 3 mg/100 ml blood (Solomon et al 1990), and ketones should not normally be found in urine unless glucose is unavailable (due either to insulin lack or starvation). Ketosis should be treated by the urgent administration of insulin.

Constipation

Constipation is frequently a problem for older people. Although physiological changes in the large intestine contribute towards constipation, more likely reasons are:

- dehydration
- low-fibre diet
- limited mobility
- drugs (e.g. narcotics and diuretics).

Gut motility is stimulated by movement. But many older people experience reduced mobility, whether from acute problems, such as a fracture, or chronic problems, such as arthritis. As well as causing discomfort, constipation further reduces appetite.

Laxatives or other aperients can be useful to resolve short-term problems with constipation, but they are unlikely to reverse the cause. In easing the passing of stools, they fail to stimulate the colonic muscle. Like any other underused muscle, the colonic muscle becomes weaker, making further episodes of constipation more likely. Therefore, whenever possible, constipation should be managed by reversing the underlying problems through:

- fluids
- fibre
- exercise.

The daily recommended fibre intake for older people is 18 grams/day (Devlin 2000).

Contrary to popular belief, most people do not open their bowels once every day (Heaton et al 1992). But, while healthcare staff usually measure constipation by frequency of bowel movement, patients may report constipation because they are straining at stool or because their stools are hard (Locke et al 2000). Therefore, when discussing problems, it is important to ensure that both staff and patients understand each other's meanings.

The central nervous system

From the age of 25 to 75, the brain's weight reduces by 10%-15% (Herbert and Thomson 1997), although intelligence and neuropsychological function do not correlate with brain size. While death of cells reduces the number of functional nerves, a lifetime's experience should mean greater use of remaining cells. Brain cells can compensate for loss of numbers by generating new synaptic connections (Herbert and Thomson 1997), and physiological reserve usually prevents loss of function despite significant cell loss. So media images of age being synonymous with dementia are grossly oversimplistic. Many people retain healthy cognitive abilities throughout life or to an advanced age. Neurological disease is not a normal consequence of ageing. Nevertheless, various mental health problems can occur, and physiological changes can cause or contribute to this process ('organic' disease).

Cell loss varies between different areas of the brain; the pons and medulla (brain stem) seem more resistant, while the hippocampus (part of the limbic system, associated with memory) is more vulnerable (Herbert and Thomson 1997). Functions controlled by areas where significant degeneration occurs will be impaired unless sufficient control can be replaced by other nerves. So many 'problems' of old age, such as reduced sensitivity to cold, reduced heat production (possible hypothermia) and changes in sleep patterns result partly from neurological changes. The autonomic nervous system, which controls most essential and basic functions of life, often shows symptomatic decline in old age (Marieb 2001), as illustrated by the discussion of baroreceptors in Chapter 4.

Pathological damage, such as atherosclerotic changes and strokes, can cause the loss of large areas of brain tissue. Senility should be considered as an unfortunate result of possible pathological processes, rather than as an inevitable part of normal ageing. Blood supply to the brain is protected by the Circle of Willis, a circular artery at the base of the brain. Being circular, obstruction from thrombi can be bypassed by the flow from the opposite direction. Owing largely to systemic arteriosclerosis, cerebral blood flow does reduce by 10%–15%, but increased dissociation of oxygen from haemoglobin provides further compensation (Herbert and Thomson 1997).

The brain relies on a constant supply of oxygen and nutrients; so an inadequate supply of either rapidly causes cerebral dysfunction. Cerebral hypoxia (e.g. caused by a chest infection) is likely to cause acute confusion. Diabetic crises (hypoglycaemia) similarly starve the brain of available nutrients and so may cause confusion. Acute confusion can also be caused by a variety of other factors, such as sensory imbalance (discussed in the next chapter). Therefore, whenever anyone appears to be confused, possible causes of acute confusion should be considered. People with a diagnosis of chronic confusional states (e.g. dementia) may also suffer from additional acute confusion.

Parkinson's disease

Parkinson's disease is a progressive disorder affecting learned voluntary movements (e.g. walking, talking, writing, swallowing), with at least half of sufferers being severely disabled (Slack 1999). It usually begins in the fifth to sixth decade of life (Marieb 2001), although a significant minority (one in seven) of sufferers develops the disease before reaching 40 (Delieu and Keady 1997). One in every hundred people over the age of 65 has Parkinson's disease, an incidence that increases to one in every fifty people over the age of 85.

Parkinson's disease is caused by insufficient cerebral production of dopamine. Dopamine is an excitatory neurotransmitter produced in the brain stem. Brain-stem homeostasis is normally maintained by balancing dopamine against the inhibitive neurotransmitter acetylcholine. Lack of dopamine therefore causes excessive nervous-system inhibition, and therefore a loss of motor control. Symptoms occur when 70–80% of dopamine-producing neurones are lost (Crabb 2000). Partial transmission of synapses may enable weakened responses, but total failure of transmission may cause 'freezing' or 'on/off' syndrome.

There are no tests to diagnose Parkinson's disease; it is either diagnosed from symptoms or at post-mortem. The cause is not always identifiable, but can include:

- drugs and chemicals (e.g. carbon monoxide, synthetic heroin, haloperidol, chlorpromazine)
- chromosome 4 defects (Youdim and Riederer 1997)
- head injuries (especially in boxers) (Delieu and Keady 1997)
- multi-infarct strokes (Delieu and Keady 1997)
- viral infections (most famously the encephalitis lethargica epidemic of 1917–1923 (Sacks 1990); although there are now few survivors from this particular epidemic).

Nerve inhibition and muscle weakness/rigidity cause the typical physical symptoms of Parkinson's disease:

- persistent tremor at rest (including head-nodding and 'pin-rolling' finger movements)
- limb rigidity (slowed movements)
- bradykinesia (e.g. shuffling gait)
- impaired balance.

Facial muscle weakness causes:

- a still (blank) facial expression
- a 'hanging' face, and dribbling
- monotonous and indistinct speech.

Weakness of other muscles can cause:

- constipation
- incontinence
- hypotension when standing upright (Goldstein et al 2000).

In an attempt to compensate for reduced muscle control and shuffling gait, people with Parkinson's tend to stoop forward when walking. This changes their centre of gravity, which, together with the other problems of walking, may result in falling.

Not everyone will suffer all symptoms; so care requires a skilful assessment of problems and needs. Rigidity may cause pain, especially at night-time (e.g. night cramps), and may cause falls or other accidents. Blank expressions may prevent obvious signs of pain. A need for pain relief and management should therefore be actively considered by healthcare staff. Gray and Hildebrand's (2000) study found that 59% of their sample experienced falls.

Parkinson's disease does not affect intelligence, although 20–60% do suffer from dementia (Delieu and Keady 1997), and many people may suffer concurrent, but unrelated, physical or mental health problems. Sleep is disturbed in 41% of women and 25% of men (Herndon et al 2000). Other people may respond to the blank expression of someone who has Parkinson's disease by assuming there is some cognitive impairment. This can be intensely frustrating to those with Parkinson's disease. Clinical depression may be organic (due to changes in the central nervous system) or reactive (in response to the physical symptoms listed above or to the way they are treated by other people). Reduced serotonin levels may contribute to organic changes (Herndon et al 2000).

As dopamine in its natural form is unable to cross the blood-brain barrier, Parkinson's disease is treated by giving the dopamine pre-cursor L-dopa, included in sinemet (carbidopa) tablets. Therefore, the dopamine infusions sometimes seen on wards will not help to alleviate the symptoms of Parkinson's disease. Although symptoms can be controlled with L-dopa (and its derivatives), there is no cure for Parkinson's disease and, being a progressive disease, increasingly higher doses of drugs are often needed. With drug control, life expectancy is normal. L-dopa has a number of significant adverse effects, including possible neurodegeneration (Marieb 2001).

Substantia nigra cells – the dopamine-producing cells of the brain stem – from both humans and animals have been transplanted into adults suffering from Parkinson's disease. These transplants appear to have been successful but incur the costs of surgery and raise ethical concerns (especially if harvested from aborted fetuses). Identification of cellular apoptosis (see Chapter 2) in the brain of a Parkinson's sufferer has led to clinical trials with anti-apoptocic drugs (Schapira 2000).

Strokes

A stroke (or cerebrovascular accident – CVA) is caused by blood failing to supply part of the brain. Brain tissue is especially susceptible to a lack of oxygen and nutrients, cells dying within two to three minutes of ischaemia (at normal body temperature) (Bickerstaff 1978). Atherosclerosis (see Chapter 4) can affect cerebral circulation as much as any other blood vessels. In older age, cerebral blood flow has reduced by 10–15%, although increased release of oxygen from haemoglobin can compensate for cerebral ischaemia (Herbert and Thomson 1997).

Traditionally, strokes are associated with hypertension. Hypertension may cause cerebral blood vessels to rupture (a bleed; typically a subarachnoid haemorrhage) or dislodge part of an arterial thrombus, thus causing an embolus. Emboli are carried along with the normal blood flow, but, once they reach vessels too small to pass through, they lodge in and obstruct further flow. Tissue beyond the obstruction is therefore deprived of blood, nutrients and oxygen and so infarcts. Strokes may also be caused by hypotension: low blood pressure results in insufficient perfusion pressure to supply tissues with nutrients and oxygen.

Strokes may range from severe, often fatal, to ones so mild they create a few transient, and potentially undetected, symptoms. A stroke causing only very brief loss of function is called a *transient ischaemic attack* (TIA). Recovery can be prolonged, and often incomplete, with disabilities ranging from mild to extensive. Nerves are rarely limited to specific functions; so movements can often be relearned through use of other nerves.

The genitourinary system

From about the age of 40, an average of 1% of nephrons are lost each year (Guyton and Hall 2000); although, in health, there is such a large functional reserve of nephrons that enough remain to last a lifetime. The glomerular surface area is reduced, and membrane thickness is increased (Clark 2000) and so the remaining nephrons become less efficient. By old age, renal blood flow reduces by up to a half (Schwertz and Buschmann 1989) due to cardiovascular problems such as systemic atherosclerosis (Clark 2000). Reduced renal blood flow reduces glomerular filtration and so the clearance of waste products. Renal tubules become shorter, so selective re-absorption (primarily of water and electrolytes) is less efficient (Clark 2000). This predisposes older people to dehydration. As with all body muscle, muscle tone is reduced. So the bladder becomes weaker and the person more likely to develop urinary incontinence.

Age-related changes also occur in the urethral tract. Whereas the female urethra is normally about 3–4 cm (Marieb 2001) and relatively straight, the male urethra is about 20 cm (Marieb 2001) and relatively convoluted. These gender differences place women at greater risk of cystitis and incontinence. With age, the female urethra becomes even shorter, and the maximum urethral closing pressure is reduced (Tobin 1992), exposing women to a greater risk of incontinence.

Incontinence is not, however, an inevitable part of growing older, to be treated by pads and catheters. However, it is a common problem and can often be reduced. Continence-promotion specialists can be a valuable source of information and advice for both staff and patients.

Cystitis may be reduced by maintaining good hygiene. After bowel movements, cleaning by wiping away from, rather than towards, the urethra, reduces transmission of bowel bacteria, especially E coli. There is some evidence that drinking cranberry juice also reduces cystitis (Fleet 1994).

Although there has usually been some earlier slight decline in reproductive function, and the risk of complications from pregnancy increase during the fourth and fifth decade of life (Herbert 1999), the menopause can cause women to undergo significant and relatively sudden physiological and psychological changes. Some physiological effects have been identified in previous chapters. Use of hormone replacement therapy is already significantly reducing the physiological effects of menopause. Following menopause, secondary sex organs atrophy. Alterations in body image from atrophy of breast tissue can compound psychological stress.

Men usually undergo a continuing decline in reproductive function, but the so-called 'male menopause' is a myth. Men continue to produce sperm, although production does decline. Other significant changes also occur to the male reproductive system. Prostate enlargement occurs in three-quarters of men over 65 (Eliopoulos 1997). As the prostate surrounds the urethra, enlargement can eventually occlude urinary flow, causing retention of urine in older men, with delay in completing voiding of the bladder ('dribbling incontinence'). The retention of urine in the bladder causes pain. Back pressure to the kidneys can cause renal infection and damage. Therefore, many older men have to undergo surgery to remove part of the prostate gland. Production of the main male hormone, testosterone, declines with age. Among other effects, testosterone increases muscle bulk. Therefore, reduced testosterone production in older age is partly responsible for muscle wasting (and weakness).

While reproductive ability may cease in women and decline in men, libido is the result of both physiological and psychological function. Libido can, and often does, survive loss of fertility. Even if physically unable to reproduce, older people may retain sexual needs, which may be very diverse. Healthcare workers caring for older people should therefore not assume that old people have lost their sexual appetites or abandoned sexual activity.

Conclusion

Ageing affects all parts of the body, to a greater or lesser extent. This chapter has described the main systems not covered in other chapters to help readers provide holistic care. Although some more-frequently encountered age-related pathologies have been included, discussion has necessarily been selective; so readers specializing in particular fields of healthcare may need to extend their knowledge further. Problems not particularly related to the ageing process, such as pain, have been excluded (there are many texts providing detailed and useful discussion of pain and its management).

Physiological health is too often taken for granted until it is lost or threatened. Knowledge of how body systems function, and how they are affected by ageing, can help healthcare workers promote physical health. However, health is more than just physiological function. The remaining chapters in this book show how health, in its widest sense, can be compromised by ageing, and how healthcare workers can help maintain the quality of life of older people.

References

Abbas A K, Lichtman A H and Pober J S (1994) Cellular and Molecular Immunology 2nd edn. Philadelphia: WB Saunders.

Bickerstaff E R (1978) Neurology 3rd edn. London: Hodder & Stoughton.

Clark B (2000) Biology of renal ageing in humans. Advances in Renal Replacement Therapy 7 (1): 11–21.

Connolly M J (1996) Obstructive airways disease: a hidden disability in the aged. Age and Ageing 25 (4): 265–267.

Crabb L (2000) Motor fluctuations in Parkinson's disease. Professional Nurse 15 (4): 273–277.

Delieu J and Keady J (1997) The biology of dementia due to Parkinson's Disease. British Journal of Nursing 6 (14): 806–810.

Devlin M (2000) The nutritional needs of the older person. Professional Nurse 16 (3): 951–955

Dunning P and Martin M (1998) Beliefs about diabetes and diabetic complications. Professional Nurse 13 (7): 429–434.

Eliopoulos C (1997) Gerontological Nursing 4th edn. Philadelphia: Lippincott.

Fleet J C (1994) New support for a folk remedy: cranberry juice reduces bacteriuria and pyuria in elderly women. Nutrition Review 52 (5): 168–170.

Goldstein D S, Holmes C, Li S-T, Bruce S, Metman L V and Cannon R O III (2000) Cardiac sympathetic denervation in Parkinson's disease. Annals of Internal Medicine 133 (5): 338–347.

Gray P and Hildebrand K (2000) Fall risk factors in Parkinson's disease. Journal of Neuroscience Nursing 32 (4): 222–228.

Guyton A C and Hall J E (2000) Textbook of Medical Physiology 10th edn. Philadelphia: W B Saunders Company.

Heaton K W, Radvan J, Cripps H, Mountford R A, Braddon F E M, Hughes A O (1992) Defecation frequency and timing, and stool form in the general population: a prospective study. Gut 33 (6): 818–824.

Herbert R A and Thomson H (1997) Biological approaches to ageing and mental health. In: Norman and I J Redfern S J (eds) Mental Health Care for Elderly People pp. 43–66. Edinburgh: Churchill Livingstone.

Herbert R A (1999) The biology of human ageing. In: Redfern S J and Ross F M (eds) Nursing Older People 3rd edn. pp. 55–77. Edinburgh: Churchill Livingstone.

Herndon C M, Young K, Herndon A D and Dole E J (2000) Parkinson's disease revisited. Journal of Neuroscience Nursing 32 (4): 216–221.

Hough A (1996) Physiotherapy in Respiratory Care. London: Chapman & Hall.

Locke G R, Pemberton J H and Phillips S P (2000) AGA technical review on constipation. Gastroenterology 119 (6): 1766–1778.

Marieb E N (2001) Human Anatomy and Physiology 5th edn. San Francisco: Benjamin/ Cummings Publishing Company Inc.

Marshall S (1996) The perioperative management of diabetes. Care of the Critically Ill 12 (2): 64–68.

Rebenson-Piano M (1989) The physiologic changes that occur with age. Critical Care Nursing Quarterly 12 (1): 1–14.

Renwick D S and Connolly M J (1995) Prevalence and treatment of chronic airways obstruction in adults over the age of 45. Thorax 51 (2): 164–168.

Rhoades R and Pflanzer P (1996) Human Physiology 3rd edn. Fort Worth: Saunders College Publishing.

Sacks O (1990) Awakenings revised edn. London: Picador.

Schapira A (2000) Parkinson's disease. Geriatric Medicine 30 (11): 39–41.

Schwertz D and Buschmann M (1989) Pharmacogeriatrics. Critical Care Nursing Quarterly 12 (1): 26–37.

Slack J (1999) Mobility. In: Heath H and Schofield I (eds) Healthy Ageing: nursing older people pp. 251–272. London: Mosby.

Solomon E P, Schmidt R R and Adragna P J (1990) Human Anatomy and Physiology 2nd edn. Fort Worth: Saunders College Publishing.

Storer J (1996) The liver. In: Hinchliff S M, Montague S E and Watson R (eds) Physiology for Nursing Practice 2nd edn. pp. 504–529. London: Baillière Tindall.

Tobin G W (1992) Incontinence in the Elderly. London: Edward Arnold.

World Health Organisation (1980) Expert Committee on Diabetes Mellitus. W H O technical report 646: 1–79.

Youdim M B H and Riederer P (1997) Understanding Parkinson's Disease. Scientific American 276 (1): 38–45.

CHAPTER 6

The special senses

PHILIP WOODROW

Introduction

Previous chapters explore the main systems promoting homeostasis. The functioning of these systems is necessary for health. But health is more than just maintaining biological homeostasis. Healthcare should promote quality of life. Quality of life includes the ability to understand, make sense of and interact with, our environment. The pathway for making sense of our environment begins with the five senses:

- sight
- hearing
- taste
- touch
- smell.

Although use differs between individuals (and some people are denied use of some senses, e.g. through blindness), most human beings use sight and hearing to a far greater extent than the other senses. Therefore, this chapter focuses on sight and hearing, with brief summaries of the other senses.

Healthy sensory function relies on:

- reception
- transmission
- perception.

Reception involves the function of receptors (e.g. taste buds). In health, signals are transmitted from receptors to the brain, which then interprets signals (perception). Sensory dysfunction can involve any one (or more) of these processes. Age-related decline in nerve function and the higher centres (cognitive function) can affect sensory health. This chapter, however, concentrates primarily on reception.

A phrase commonly used about computers is 'garbage in, garbage out'. For a computer to make sense of information, the information itself must make sense. Similarly, the brain relies on receiving reliable information. If information is inaccurate, imbalanced or absent, the brain is likely to make abnormal interpretations (e.g. hallucinations, delusions). Many factors can cause imbalanced sensory inputs, including reduced-sensory receptors and a degeneration of nerve pathways.

Many anatomical names of parts of sensory organs are not widely used outside specialist areas. Where the use of anatomical names could obscure the meaning, colloquial names are also given.

Sight

For most people, sight is the most important sense. Eye contact forms a significant component of communication, especially associated with friendliness and honesty (Niven 2000). Therefore, in addition to the obvious physiological complications from impaired vision, eye and sight problems can affect a person's social life. Almost one million people in the UK are registered as being blind; most of these are aged over 65 (Clisby and Cox 1999).

External structures

The eye is particularly delicate and so is protected by various external structures, including a socket of bone. With age, the loss of periorbital fat causes eye recession (Herbert 1999), creating the potentially eerie appearance of sunken eyes.

Various muscles surround the eye. Like other muscles (see Chapter 3), eye muscles usually weaken with age, limiting eye movement in older people. However, various other age-related changes are likely to cause greater problems for older people. The loss of the elastic tissue of the eyebrow and upper lid can cause ptosis and occlusion of the upper-visual field (Herbert 1999). The loss of the elastic tissue in the lower lid may allow it to fall forwards, causing the lid to separate from the eye (Herbert 1999), which prevents the normal drainage of tears. The tear ducts may also become blocked. Either of these problems will cause epiphora ('watery eyes'), a particularly common condition among older people (Allan 1996).

Tears

Tears are secreted by lacrimal glands and spread by the blink reflex. Blinking occurs (usually subconsciously) several times each minute. This spreads a thin (10-micrometre) film over the surface of the eye. Excess tears drain into the nasal cavity, which is why we often need to blow our nose when crying. Tears are mainly a dilute saline solution but also contain a number of protective factors, including:

- mucus
- antibodies
- lysozyme.

Antibodies and lysozyme are part of the non-specific immune system and so help protect the eye from infection. Tear production declines with age, making older people more prone to the drying of eye surfaces, corneal damage and eye infections. Post-menopausal women are especially prone to developing dry eyes (Lueckenotte 2000).

Infection

The surface of the eye is particularly susceptible to infection. The most common infecting organisms are streptococcus, staphylococcus aureus and haemophilic influenza (Fox 1989). Surface bacteria may cause the inflammation of eyelash follicles and sebaceous glands (blepharitis). Blepharitis makes the eye red, swollen and sore, with crusts of dried mucus collecting on the eyelids. These crusts may cause corneal damage as blinking draws the eyelid (and crusts) over the corneal surface.

Internal structure

The eye has two main parts, separated by the lens. The part in front of the lens has two chambers: the anterior chamber between the cornea and the iris, and the posterior chamber between the iris and the lens. Both chambers in front of the lens are filled with watery 'aqueous humour'. Behind the lens is a thicker, jelly-like 'vitreous humour' or 'vitreous body'. Vitreous humour is formed during fetal life and lasts through life. Aqueous humour is secreted from the ciliary processes near the lens. About 2–3 microlitres of aqueous humour is secreted every minute, flowing through the anterior chamber and draining through the canal of Schlemm into the extra-ocular venous blood (Guyton and Hall 2000).

Anything obstructing this flow through the canal of Schlemm, such as blood cells and tissue debris from an intra-ocular haemorrhage, causes relatively rapid accumulation of aqueous humour within the anterior chamber. This increases intra-ocular pressure, which in turn compresses the retina and the ocular nerve.

Blood vessels in front of the retina would impair vision; so ocular blood supply ends at the capillaries on the retina. Vitreous and aqueous humours, therefore, not only fill the eyeball, helping it to retain its shape, but also supply oxygen and nutrients to the eye tissues. Just as blood exerts a pressure on the blood-vessel walls ('blood pressure'), so the ocular humours place pressure on the surfaces of the eye ('intra-ocular pressure'). Normal intra-ocular pressure is about 15 mmHg (Guyton and Hall 2000). Raised intra-ocular pressure causes papilloedema (seen through an ophthalmoscope as a bulge on the optic disc, where the retina and optic nerve meet). Excessive pressure damages the nerve. Sustained pressures above 20–30 mmHg, or short periods (potentially as little as a few minutes) of 60–70 mmHg, may cause blindness.

Glaucoma

Glaucoma (ocular nerve damage) is characterized by:

- elevated intra-ocular pressure
- optic-nerve injury
- visual loss.

Glaucoma is slowly progressive, eventually causing blindness. About 250,000 people in the UK have glaucoma, most of whom are either middle-aged or older (IGA 2000). It is a possible complication of diabetes.

Conjunctiva

The eyelid and sclera (the unseen part of the eyeball) are covered by conjunctiva, a mucous membrane. This lubricates the eye surface, providing a barrier against anything from the environment that might harm the eye. In health, the conjunctival membrane is transparent.

In older people the cornea and conjunctiva often become thinner (Herbert 1999). But the conjunctiva can also become inflamed (*conjunctivitis*). Bleeding from the very delicate blood vessels of the conjunctiva causes eyes to become red ('redeye', 'bloodshot'). Inflammation may be due to viral or bacterial infection.

Cornea

Not having a direct blood supply, the cornea, which is exposed to the environment, is particularly susceptible to infection. Eye infections are therefore highly contagious. Being on the surface of the eye, the cornea is at risk of traumatic damage (e.g. from overvigorous rubbing of eyes). Corneal ulceration exposes deeper tissues within the eye to bacteria from the environment. A lack of a regular blood supply makes repair slow, and potentially incomplete (permanent visual impairment). The cornea has a rich nerve supply; so lacerations are usually very painful.

Lens and iris

The iris, separating the anterior from the posterior chambers, contains the pupil and the muscles. The muscles control the size of the pupil and so the amount of light reaching visual receptors. Although the pupil normally dilates when light is reduced and constricts when light is increased, the muscles are controlled by both sympathetic and parasympathetic nerves; so anything affecting nerve signals (e.g. morphine) affects pupil dilation. With age, the iris becomes more fibrous, reducing the pupil's ability to dilate and so reducing the amount of light reaching visual receptors in the retina (Herbert 1999).

Throughout life, the lens becomes progressively more dense, more convex and less elastic. As a result, images reaching the retina change (Allan 1996), near vision is lost and there is greater difficulty in focusing on objects (Herbert 1999). The inability to focus due to reduced lens elasticity is called 'presbyopia'. Typically, sight problems change with age from being short-sighted to long-sighted. 'Short' and 'long' sighted refer to whether images fall 'short' (i.e. before) or 'long' (i.e. after) the retina, and, while short-sighted and near-vision (or long-sighted and distance-vision) often occur at the same time, they are not necessarily synonymous. Age-related changes in the shape of lenses reduce the amount of light reaching the retina; so older people often need more light for reading (Herbert 1999).

Cataracts

As the lens hardens and thickens, it becomes more opaque ('cataract'), causing the vision to be cloudy and reducing the ability to distinguish colours (Clisby and Cox 1999). Although cataracts can occur at any age, they become especially common in old age, more than 60% occurring in people over 85 years of age (Tuft 2000). In the West, they are the main cause of blindness in people over 65 (Armbrecht et al 2000). Diabetes mellitus increases the risk of developing cataracts. People living in inner cities are also more likely to develop cataracts (Tuft 2000). Other factors, such as smoking and exposure to intensive sunlight, have also been linked to cataract development (Marieb 2001). Cataracts can be surgically removed, and over 160,000 cataracts are removed each year in the UK (Tuft 2000).

Retina

The retina, at the back of the eye, has two layers, one containing the vision-receptor cells (cones and rods) and the other the beginnings of the ocular nerves. The age-related loss of the receptors in the retina reduces the size of the visual field (Herbert 1999).

These two layers of the retina can separate (*retinal detachment*). Separation allows vitreous humour to seep between them. Surgical replacement can save the person's vision, but, if not replaced, the retina is eventually destroyed, causing permanent blindness.

Implications for practice

Loss of, or impaired, vision removes the main sense used by most people. Items that are likely to be needed should be placed nearby, and the person told or shown where they are. Guiding the person's hand to touch each object is a useful way to 'show' visually impaired people. Some form of bell or alarm should be within easy reach. Products such as large-print books and audio books can improve the quality of life for many people with impaired vision. Hospital and nursing-home signs normally use large print, but in other places (e.g. hotels) more explanations may be needed of where facilities are.

Environmental safety should be ensured. People with a new visual impairment should be orientated within their environment. Some risk factors can be replaced, such as rucks in rugs and carpets, although changes to the person's own home or property should respect their autonomy and right to choose. Risk factors that cannot be removed should be identified, either by explanation or by 'showing' the person (often through the use of touch). Mobility and safety factors may need to be assessed by occupational therapists and physiotherapists.

As well as supplying glasses, opticians can identify various visual problems that may benefit from further medical attention, such as glaucoma. People wearing glasses should have their sight checked regularly (usually every two years). Glasses should be clean and fit well. If glasses are broken, they should be repaired or replaced by an optician. Amateur repairs with tape should not be used, as this may cause misalignment of the lenses, and possible adaptive damage to the eye.

Hearing

Air conducts light better than it conducts sound. While light travels at 186,000 miles per second, sound travels only at 0.2 miles per second (Marieb 2001), hence the difference in time between seeing lightning and hearing thunder. Sound travels far better through a more solid medium that can transmit sound waves; so, whereas sound travels at 344 metres per second in air, fresh water of 20°C transmits it at 1450 metres per second (Ganong 1999). The human ear provides such a medium to enable sound to travel quickly. The ear comprises three main parts:

- outer
- middle
- inner.

The outer ear

The outer ear consists of the:

- auricle (or pinna)
- external auditory canal
- tympanic membrane.

The auricle, which is cartilage covered by a thin layer of skin, directs sound waves into the ear. The external auditory canal is the short chamber connecting the auricle to the tympanic membrane. It contains sebaceous and modified-apocrine sweat glands. Sebaceous glands lubricate the skin (see Chapter 3). Ceruminous glands, modified sweat glands, secrete cerumen ('ear wax'). Cerumen is often viewed as a nuisance, and (especially for older people) it can be. But it does have important physiological functions: trapping foreign bodies (keeping the ear clear) and repelling insects (Marieb 2001). When cerumen dries it should fall out naturally. But accumulated wax can block the auditory canal, and so impair hearing. The number of ceruminous and sebaceous glands decreases with age (Bennett and Ebrahim 1995), and cerumen becomes harder and less likely to clear (Coni et al 1993); one in four older people suffers from plugs of cerumen and dry, scaly skin (Herbert 1991).

The tympanic membrane ('ear drum') is a thin, translucent membrane of connective tissue. Sound waves hitting the tympanum initiate vibrations, which travel into the inner ear. With age, the tympanic membrane thickens. Thicker materials vibrate less, impairing sound conduction.

Accumulated ear wax, impairing hearing, tempts some people to try to remove it with solid objects. These solid objects may rupture the very delicate tympanum. A torn drum will not vibrate; so, if earwax does need to be removed, it should be done carefully using a flannel or soft cloth soaked in warm water, which should remove sufficient wax. If this fails, an experienced and qualified person should syringe the ear.

Middle ear

Immediately behind the tympanic membrane is the tympanic cavity. Like any drum, the eardrum needs a pocket of air to resonate. The eardrum will only vibrate if pressure is equal on both sides. So the Eustachian (or 'pharyngotympanic' or 'auditory') tube connects the middle ear with the nasopharynx. Normally, this tube is flat and closed, but, when yawning, coughing or swallowing, it opens to equalize pressures on both sides of the membrane (Ganong 1999) (hence the use of boiled sweets by some airlines). When the tube is blocked (e.g. by viral infections, such as colds), pressures on each side of the tympanic membrane differ, the membrane bulges and sound is poorly transmitted. This impairs hearing and may cause earache.

The middle ear is a small area spanned by three connected bones called either by their Latin or English names: malleus ('hammer'), incus ('anvil') and stapes ('stirrup'). These bones are very small, but very important. Because they are interlinked, but moveable, they transmit vibrations of sound from the tympanic membrane to the oval window of the inner ear. These auditory ossicles amplify sound twentyfold (van de Graaff et al. 1997). With age, movement of these bones becomes progressively less sensitive, affecting the localization of sound (Walker 1989). So even if older people hear a sound, they may not be sure where it is from, or be able to identify who is speaking to them.

Inner ear

The inner ear, or labyrinth, is filled with perilymph and endolymph. Despite their names, these are derived from cerebrospinal fluid (CSF), not lymph (Marieb 2001). This fluid makes a good medium for the transmission of sound. The inner ear has three parts:

- vestibule
- cochlea
- semicircular canals.

Near the cochlea are the semicircular canals, which control balance. Therefore, problems with the middle ear (e.g. infection) can affect balance, potentially resulting in falls.

The cochlea is very small, but crucial to hearing. Inside the cochlea is the organ of Corti, containing hairs that act as auditory receptors. At birth there are some 40,000 hairs in the cochlea (Marieb 2001). Sound waves transmitted through fluid move these hairs, stimulating nerves at their bases. These impulses are then transmitted through the cochlear nerve, a branch of the vestibulocochlear nerve (cranial nerve VIII), into the central nervous system, where messages are interpreted (perceived) in the temporal lobe.

Although ageing affects all parts of the ear, age-related changes in the inner ear are particularly detrimental to hearing (Luxon 1993). Cochleal hairs are progressively lost and not replaced through life. Marieb (2001) suggests that by the age of 140 no hairs would remain. Tinnitus, a constant ringing in the ears, can be caused by a degeneration of the cochlear nerve, although there are many other causes. Tinnitus is a relatively common age-related problem, occurring in 13–44% of older people (Luxon 1993).

Hearing loss (*presbyacusis*)

Hearing loss may be either conductive or sensorineural. Conductive hearing loss is where the mechanisms that transmit sound are impaired (e.g. thickening of the tympanic membrane), whereas sensorineural hearing loss is caused by an impairment of the nervous system (usually a dysfunction of the cochlea or cochlear nerve, but sometimes from central nervous system dysfunction (Fook and Morgan 2000)). The ability to perceive sound is best at about 10 years of age (Herbert 1999). Hearing usually then degenerates, with particular loss of higher pitches. Ninety per cent of people with hearing loss of 45 decibels are over 52 years of age (Fook and Morgan 2000), and one-third of people aged 60–70 have hearing impairment (Le May 1999a).

Consonants have a higher frequency (Bennett and Ebrahim 1995) and so are more likely to be unclear. Sounds particularly affected by hearing loss are those ranging between 2000 and 8000 vibrations per second: S, SH, F, TH, CH, D, T (Levene 1985). Were one to choose any paragraph from any text (e.g. newspaper, magazine) and counted how often these sounds occurred, one would see how difficult they are to avoid. S is the second most frequently used letter in the English language (e being the most frequent); it is almost impossible to avoid in any sentence, but the use of s can consciously be reduced – using singular rather than plural words limits the number of s's.

Cognitive problems (confusion, dementia) compound the perceptual difficulties of hearing. So older people are more likely to have difficulty hearing and understanding what is said to them. Hearing problems may also be compounded by ototoxic drugs (such as gentamicin). Hearing difficulties effectively increase isolation (Gilhome Herbst 1999), and may exacerbate mental health problems, such as paranoia (Woods and Birren 1998).

Implications for practice

A number of simple, but important, strategies can improve perception of hearing, all of which centre around making the most of remaining sensory pathways. Too often the strategy adopted for deafness is to shout louder. This is effectively what a hearing aid does – it amplifies the volume. The effect of shouting can be experienced by listening to a radio that is out of tune. Turning up the volume makes the noise louder, not clearer, and may even become painful. People may respond angrily if they are shouted at. Shouting is therefore one common strategy that should be avoided.

Watching someone's lip movements and facial expression assists communication (Wright 1988). So, when speaking to older people, try to face them and be within comfortable viewing distance. If the person normally wears glasses, they should be in place and clean.

Various visual aids can help people with impaired hearing maintain independence, for example visual doorbells and telephones. Many places of entertainment, such as theatres, have hearing loops to help the hard of hearing maintain a good quality of life. Social clubs and support groups can similarly help prevent social isolation.

With the loss of higher-frequency sounds, lower voices will probably be heard more clearly, as well as being more comforting (Feil 1993). Slower speech is easier to follow (Gilhome Herbst 1999), will tend to be lower and is the easiest strategy to adopt for hearing and/or cognitive impairment. Talking to someone with hearing impairment requires a skilled balancing of recognizing their needs without being patronising. Remembering what it is like to try to understand a different language can be a useful reminder of others' needs. Possible distractions should be minimized: background television or radio should, if possible, be turned off or down when speaking to someone. Repeating or rephrasing what is being said may help understanding.

Hearing aids

Hearing aids are available for chronic hearing impairment. About one-quarter of old people will benefit from, and accept, a hearing aid (Coni et al 1993). Despite limitations, hearing aids do help many people with hearing problems, but owners of hearing aids may have bad experiences in hospitals. If unable to look after the aid themselves (e.g. arthritis may rob them of the manual dexterity needed to change the batteries and adjust the settings), people rely on others to help them. Like any other personal possession, hearing aids should be looked after, not lost or broken. Most hearing aids are now the behind-the-ear (BTE) design, which should be placed in the ear for which they are made. Function should be checked regularly, and dead batteries replaced promptly. Whistles from hearing aids are likely to irritate both the wearer and others.

Hearing aids prevent cerumen from falling out, and provide a surface for it to adhere to. Ears should be inspected regularly for cerumen accumulation, and cleaned according to local guidelines. Hearing aids should also be inspected and cleaned regularly (Fountain 1987) (at least once a day). Anyone wearing a hearing aid should be under the care of an audiologist. Staff working in long-stay areas should involve audiologists as part of the care team for anyone wearing a hearing aid.

Touch

Of the three remaining senses, touch is usually the most-used one. Touch significantly contributes to non-verbal communication, becoming especially important for people with visual impairment.

With age, the number of touch receptors diminishes, while impaired nerve function slows the transmission of tactile messages. The sense of touch, therefore, becomes less sensitive in older age. In addition, pathological damage, such as a stroke, can partially or totally destroy nerve pathways from certain parts of the body. Peripheral neuropathy is a complication especially associated with diabetes mellitus.

Implications for practice

Touch is a valuable sense both for protection and to replace visual loss. Therefore, impaired tactile senses prevent the warning signals of tissue damage. For example, people sitting near a fire or using a hot water bottle may be exposing part of their skin to prolonged heat, but, not sensing any pain, do not change their position, and so develop skin burns and blisters.

Touch helps communication. A held hand can add much to words. Touch should, however, be used positively, remembering that what feels acceptable for both staff and patients will alter with each person (Boyek and Watson 1994). Unwanted touch should never be forced on anyone (Feil 1993). From a legal perspective, touch without consent is battery, and the fear of being touched without consent is assault (Dimond 1995).

Taste

There are four types of taste:

- salt
- sweet
- sour
- bitter.

Young adults have 3000–10,000 taste buds (Guyton and Hall 2000). About four-fifths of taste is derived from smell (Marieb 2001); so the olfactory changes identified below will affect taste. The number of taste buds declines after the age of 45 (Guyton and Hall 2000). By 80 years of age, some two-thirds of taste buds may be lost (Herbert 1999), especially salt and sweet taste buds (on the tip of the tongue) (Le May 1999b). The loss of taste buds reduces the ability to distinguish between different tastes, which reduces the appeal of food and the motivation to eat. Salivary production also declines with age, which reduces the exposure of tastes to the remaining buds (Allan 1996).

People may have to change their diet for health, economical or other reasons. For example, people with dental or swallowing problems may be encouraged to take a soft diet, which often means a bland diet. Similarly, people who are unable to cook, or experience difficulty with preparing their own meals, are more likely to rely on meals provided by voluntary or other services, which often lack the flavour of freshly cooked home-prepared meals.

Implications for practice

Reduced sense of taste and/or difficulties with eating create a disincentive to eating, which might encourage malnutrition. Nutritional advice should be offered. Dietitians are a valuable resource both in the community and within hospitals. Clear but simple, printed health information, which people can reread at their leisure, is useful.

In an attempt to compensate for taste loss, people may add more flavourings to their meals. Two of the most widely available flavourings are sugar and salt, both of which may cause health problems if taken in excess. People with impaired renal function may develop oedema from additional salt intake, while reduced pancreatic function may cause extra sugar to remain in the blood stream. Health advice should include warnings against the excessive use of salt or sugar.

Smell

Olfactory receptors line the nasal cavity. As air is breathed in, the shape of the nasal cavity creates air turbulence, forcing it to circulate a number of times over the receptors before passing further down the airway. This system creates efficient exposure of smells to the olfactory receptors. It is debateable whether or not the sense of smell declines with age (Niven 2000), but age-related reduction in olfactory receptors and nerve pathways is at least possible. Eliopoulos (1997) suggests that by 80 years of age a person's sense of smell has deteriorated by half.

Many old people experience breathing problems and chronic respiratory disease. In an attempt to increase air intake, they often resort to partial mouth breathing. While this may supplement air volume, there are no olfactory receptors in the mouth for smells to be exposed to. So mouth breathing reduces the sense of smell.

Implications for practice

Smell significantly contributes towards taste; so a reduced sense of smell is likely to decrease the appetite. An impaired sense of smell can expose older people to dangers, such as failing to detect leaking gas. Their quality of life may also indirectly be affected. For example, the person may not detect, and so not remove, offensive odours from their home. These offensive odours may discourage visitors and so increase social isolation.

Sensory imbalance

The senses provide information to understand our environment. Limitation of sensory input means that only a limited sense will be made of the environment. The more gaps that exist, the more imagination has to fill those gaps. So what might internally make sense to the person may externally appear to others as confusion. The poorer the range and quality of sensory input, the more isolated from reality the person is likely to be. Sensory impairment is more likely to increase with age; so staff should individually assess each person, considering their abilities, limitations and needs.

When caring for someone who appears to be confused, carers should consider whether environmental stressors or sensory limitations have contributed to confusion. Reversing sensory imbalance can be difficult. Adopting a reality-orientation approach can be counterproductive, as it can create conflict between the confused person and the orientator. Feil's (1993) approach of Validation Therapy may prove more constructive.

There are many voluntary groups that can provide information and help for people. Some of these groups may be national (such as the Royal National Institute for the Blind) while others may be local. Healthcare workers can usefully involve these groups in care, both for their own information and to the direct benefit of their clients.

Conclusion

Isolation caused by sensory limitations will be compounded by any limitations to communication, such as dysphasia (e.g. from a stroke or Parkinson's disease). Although their cognitive abilities may be intact, other people can react in intolerant or patronizing ways, which is likely to cause frustration. Individualized assessment should identify the person's abilities so that those caring for people with any sensory impairment can optimize the use of their remaining senses (Feil 1993). Sight is the main sense used by most people and so should be used when possible to supplement hearing. Touch becomes a particularly valuable sense when both sight and hearing are impaired.

Sensory impairments can increase financial expenditure. For example, people with visual impairments may be forced to rely more on public and other transport. Some public transport systems are free to pensioners, but, where financial help is needed, staff should involve social workers.

Although social values are changing, loss or impairment of one or more senses can be a source of stigmatization, as can be seen by handicaps being a target for some forms of humour. The loss of one or more senses also threatens the individual identity and independence of the person. Therefore, there may be understandable reluctance to admit any deficits. Healthcare workers should explore these issues sensitively, including using their own observations when making individualized assessment. Health education should identify each person's needs and possible sources of help. However, the individuality and independence of each person should be respected and encouraged. Help should be offered sensitively, without treating the person as being incapable.

This chapter concludes the discussion of physiological ageing. Some application has been made to healthcare practice, but further application can, and should, be made by clinical staff according to specific individual needs. Whether the possible degenerative changes discussed will cause health problems depends on various factors, including physiological reserve and individual values and beliefs. Human beings are more than just the sum of physiological systems. Their personalities and individualities are also formed by psychological and social factors, such as those discussed in the remainder of this book. Staff need a working knowledge of physiology, but, as with any other aspect of knowledge, this should be applied to meet the individual needs of the whole person they are working with and caring for.

References

Allan D (1996) The special senses. In: Hinchliff S M, Montague S E and Watson R (eds) Physiology for Nursing Practice 2nd edn. pp. 153–184. London: Baillière Tindall.

Armbrecht A M, Findlay C, Kaushal S, Aspinall P, Hill A R, Dhillon B (2000) Is cataract surgery justified in patients with age related macular degeneration? A visual function and quality of life assessment. British Journal of Ophthalmology 84 (12): 1343–1348.

Bennett G J and Ebrahim S (1995) Healthcare in Old Age 2nd edn. London: Edward Arnold.

Boyek K and Watson R (1994) A touching story. Elderly Care 6 (3): 20–21.

Clisby C and Cox C E (1999) Sight. In: Redfern S J and Ross F M (eds) Nursing Older People 3rd edn. pp. 303–313. Edinburgh: Churchill Livingstone.

Coni N, Davison W and Webster S (1993) Lecture Notes on Geriatrics 4th edn. Oxford: Blackwell Science.

Dimond B (1995) Legal Aspects of Nursing 2nd edn. London: Prentice Hall.

Eliopoulos C (1997) Gerontological Nursing 4th edn. Philadelphia: Lippincott.

Feil N (1993) The Validation Breakthrough. Baltimore: Health Professionals Press.

Fook L and Morgan R (2000) Hearing impairment in older people: a review. Postgraduate Medical Journal 76 (899): 537–541.

Fountain D (1987) Hearing aids and their care. Geriatric Nursing and Home Care 7 (1): 12–14.

Fox J (1989) Conjunctivitis, keratitis and iritis. Nursing 3 (45): 20–23

Ganong W F (1999) Review of Medical Physiology 19th edn. Connecticut: Appleton & Lange.

Gilhome Herbst K (1999) Hearing. In: Redfern S J and Ross F M (eds) Nursing Older People 3rd edn. pp. 291–302. Edinburgh: Churchill Livingstone.

Guyton A C and Hall J E (2000) Textbook of Medical Physiology 10th edn. Philadelphia: WB Saunders Company.

Herbert R A (1991) The biology of human ageing. In: Redfern S J and Ross F M (eds) Nursing Older People 3rd edn. pp. 39–63. Edinburgh: Churchill Livingstone.

Herbert R A (1999) The biology of human ageing. In: Redfern S J and Ross F M (eds) Nursing Older People 3rd edn. pp. 55–77. Edinburgh: Churchill Livingstone.

IGA (2000) Why people over 40 should have their eyes tested for glaucoma. Fact Sheet L07 793. London: International Glaucoma Association. www.iga.org.uk/fs_107.htm

Le May A C (1999a) Communication skills. In: Redfern S J and Ross F M (eds) Nursing Older People 3rd edn. pp. 283–290. Edinburgh: Churchill Livingstone.

Le May A (1999b) Sensory and perceptual issues of ageing. In: Heath H and Schofield I (eds) Healthy Ageing: nursing older people pp. 273–195. London: Mosby.

Levene B (1985) Sensory loss in the elderly. Nursing 41 (2): 1221–1225.

Lueckenotte AG (2000) Gerontologic Nursing 2nd edn. St Louis: Mosby.

Luxon L (1993) Disorders of hearing and balance. Reviews in Clinical Gerontology 3 (4): 347–358.

Marieb E N (2001) Human Anatomy and Physiology 5th edn. San Francisco: Benjamin/Cummings Publishing Company Inc.

Niven N (2000) Health Psychology for Health Care Professionals. Edinburgh: Churchill Livingstone.

Tuft S J (2000) Cataract. Medicine 28 (9): 16–19.

Van de Graaff K M, Fox S I and Lafleur K M (1997) Synopsis of Human Anatomy & Physiology. Dubuque Ia: Wm C Brown Publishers.

Walker D (1989) Normal ageing. Nursing 3 (37): 5–8.

Woods A M and Birren J E (1998) Psychology. In: Pathy M S J (ed) Principles and Practice of Geriatric Medicine 3rd edn. pp. 55–64. Chichester: Wiley.

Wright S (1988) Communicating. In: Wright S G (ed) Nursing the Older Patient pp. 61–84. London: Chapman & Hall.

PART 2
PSYCHOLOGICAL

CHAPTER 7

Psychology and ageing

NICKY HAYES AND HENRY A MINARDI

Introduction

Ask yourself the question 'How do I feel in myself: my personality, thinking, memory, compared with how I felt ten, twenty or more years ago'.

One of the authors (NH) has informally asked this question, as part of a lecture on the psychology of ageing to successive groups of nursing students, aged between twenty and fifty, over the past three years. Most students say that they are the same person, they do not feel any different except that they think that their memory is getting worse. When pressed to explain this complaint, they usually say that they sometimes forget where they put things, they go to the shop and forget to pick up a grocery or when at work they have to write lists of tasks in case they forget to do them. They are anticipating a decline in memory even when aged less than thirty!

Memory lapses are nothing unusual at any age, and may even be interpreted with humour on occasions such as accidentally putting a knife in the fridge rather than the cutlery drawer. A forgotten grocery item is not a matter for fuss, and can be picked up later. As for forgetting something at work – nurses have a large amount of information to remember, it is not surprising if something is forgotten. However, if the person were 70 or 80 years old, at home, no longer working, these memory lapses might not be laughed off so easily. A relative or neighbour might become concerned that this person is getting forgetful – perhaps becoming a risk to themselves. Alzheimer's might even be suspected. Memory problems assume a different significance in old age.

It could be argued that negative stereotypes of ageing, such as forgetfulness, contribute to a lack of tolerance of behaviours in old people which are accepted in younger people. Older people, when depressed, sometimes reinforce the stereotype of inevitable decline by rating their memory to be worse than it is (McGlone et al 1990, Rabbitt and Abson 1990, Bolla et al 1991, Flicker et al 1993). In this chapter, it will be established that, while psychological changes do occur in later life, decline is not global, rapid or inevitable and people do retain the capacity for development in later life. This will be demonstrated by identifying and comparing the key features of some of the developmental and sociological theories of ageing. The authors' model of factors influencing psychological development in later life will then be introduced and discussed with reference to the theories. Overall, a balanced perspective on normal psychological ageing will be presented.

Outline of general models and theories from developmental psychology

Erikson

Erikson (1964) views development as an interplay between biological, social and individual development factors, with identity continuing to develop throughout life. The life span is seen as a series of stages, characterized by conflict at each stage. These are summarized in Box 7.1.

In old age, the conflict to be resolved is between what Erikson called (ego) integrity vs. despair; its resolution being the quality of wisdom. Ego integrity can be seen as an acceptance that the person's life is nearing its end, with a sense of completion of life goals and potentials. Despair is

---

Box 7.1: Erikson's stages of life

Stage	Conflict	Resolution
Infancy	Trust vs. Mistrust	Hope
Early Childhood	Autonomy vs. shame and doubt	Will
Play age	Initiative vs. guilt	Purpose
School age	Industry vs. inferiority	Competence
Adolescence	Identity vs. role confusion	Fidelity
Young adulthood	Intimacy vs. isolation	Love
Maturity	Generativity vs. stagnation	Care
Old age	Integrity vs. despair	Wisdom

From: Erikson 1964

described by Erikson as 'the petty disgust of feeling finished and passed by and the despair of facing the period of relative helplessness which marks the end as it marked the beginning' (Erikson 1964 p. 134).

The third age and activity theory

Activity theory suggests that, by maintaining activity levels into old age or replacing them with new ones, old age may be denied and life satisfaction enhanced (see Havighurst 1963): 'Use it or lose it' as the saying goes. Activity theory can be likened to the aspirations evoked by the concept of the 'third age', which is described by Laslett (1989) as an era of personal fulfilment. Young and Schuller (1983 p. 268) go further in describing the third age as a time of life when: 'older people having a certain kind of freedom – a negative freedom from coercion – which they may or may not convert into another kind of freedom, the positive kind: freedom from work'.

These views of old age offer a positive vision of fulfilment of the individual's potential and maintenance of activity. Stereotypes of old age are directly challenged; there is no place for forgetfulness and decline, at least until the fourth age is reached. The activity theory and third age views, while positive, may be criticized on several points:

- they are idealistic
- some older people may not be able to maintain activity levels because of ill health or lack of motivation
- opportunity for some activities may require a degree of prosperity that is not available to all old people
- the views take a Western perspective and may not apply to all cultures.

As a developmental approach, these views differ from Erikson's in a number of ways, particularly regarding conflict resolution, and in that Erikson does not distinguish between early old age (third age) and late old age (fourth age).

Disengagement theory

'Disengagement is an inevitable process in which many of the relationships between a person and other members of society are severed and those remaining are altered in quality' (Cumming and Henry 1961 p. 211).

This theory suggests that in old age disengagement of the individual from society occurs alongside disengagement of society from the individual.

In other words, society and the individual prepare themselves for death, which is the ultimate disengagement. Roles such as worker and parent are changed and lost in old age and not replaced. Criticism of this theory, however, has been summed up by Coleman (1993) as:

- social disengagement is not universal
- disengagement tends to be related to losses and stresses connected with age
- those who remain active and socially integrated have been shown to have a greater degree of life satisfaction than those who did disengage.

Disengagement theory can also be criticized on the grounds that it may reinforce the stereotypes of old age as a period of decline when people no longer have a valued contribution to make in society. On the other hand, if interpreted positively, it suggests that old age may be a period of reflection and allow people new freedom from social responsibilities. Coleman (1993) suggests that disengagement theory is an interesting example of both the power and danger of theories.

Levinson

Levinson (1980) likens key components of life, such as marriage, family, occupation, religion and leisure activities, to threads that run through the individual's life, with some of these threads being more central than others. Like Erikson, he saw the life cycle as a series of stages or eras, with key tasks associated with each era:

1. Childhood and adolescence
2. Early adulthood
3. Middle adulthood
4. Late adulthood.

The theory suggests that in the transition to late adulthood the person has to adjust to the idea of retirement, deal with the awareness of bodily decline and come to terms with the proximity of death. Levinson saw this as a time of development as well as decline.

The shared concept underlying these theories is one of life being a series of stages, with development occurring in some way throughout. Even the most negatively framed theory – disengagement theory – suggests that old age may be a time for reflection and freedom from social constraints. At the other extreme, activity theory advocates a proactive and liberated old age, with denial of decline and other negative consequences of old age. While these theories offer general explanations of the process of ageing, they do not necessarily reflect diversity within the population of older people: individuals will inevitably present exceptions to these theories. For this reason, the next section moves towards an individual level by outlining a model of the factors influencing individual psychological development.

Factors influencing psychological development

An overall agreement has been reached in psychology that both genetic predisposition and environmental factors affect differences and development (Atkinson et al 1996). These differences are more easily detected from childhood to young adulthood, a development that is more rapid than in old age. However, a person of 70 years would not have lost genetic influences that existed at 20 years of age. Also, because a 70-year-old has had more experiences than a 20-year-old it can safely be assumed that the environment will have a stronger influence on the older person's growth and development.

Thus, heredity and the environment are both influential in the psychological development of individuals from birth to old age. Within these two paradigms are a number of influencing factors. These have been identified by the authors as: physical health, physical environment, cognitive processes, individual differences, relationships, social and financial factors, education, and culture and ethnicity (Figure 7.1). Each of these factors has both an individual and combined influence on the psychological development of an older person. A comprehensive discussion of these factors now follows.

Physical health

There are a number of physiological changes that normally occur during the ageing process, and these can have an effect on cognitive functioning in some older people. There is considerable variation between individuals, and it has been suggested that up to 10 per cent of people may not experience cognitive decline at all, except perhaps in extreme old age (Coleman 1993). When cognitive decline does occur, an individual may still age 'successfully' and enjoy a good quality of life. In addition to 'normal' changes with age, an increase in chronic disease and acute illness may affect a person's overall sense of well-being, quality of life and cognitive function.

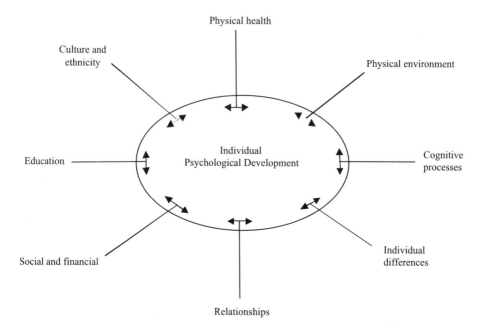

Figure 7.1: Factors influencing psychological development in later life.

Holland and Rabbitt (1991) identify the main physiological changes that affect cognitive function in old age as: an increase in blood pressure, a reduction in cerebral blood flow and changes in the levels of neuro-transmitters and glucose metabolism. These are 'normal' changes, but in some cases, influenced by pathology, cognitive decline may result. For example, although blood pressure does tend to rise with age, abnormal hypertension has been shown to be associated with substantial decline in intelligence scores in older people (Wilkie and Eisdorfer 1971). There is evidence that pathologies that reduce cerebral blood flow, such as chronic obstructive pulmonary disease and cardiovascular disease, are also predictors of cognitive decline (Grant et al 1982, Schaie 1990).

Other physiological processes and pathology that might affect cognition

There is some evidence that the decreased levels of the hormone oestrogen can have an effect on cognitive function in post-menopausal women (Sherwin 1997). For example, there may be a link between lower-circulating oestrogen, depression and anxiety, although it is not yet clear whether this is an area of health that would benefit clinically from medical intervention.

The overall contribution of physical health to psychological well-being and quality of life

Some physical health factors are important in maintaining cognitive ability and are potentially modifiable. These include physical activity, smoking, diet and, by implication, cardiovascular and pulmonary function. Physical and mental health are closely related and it is not surprising that Grundy et al (1997) found that poor physical and mental health were associated with a poor quality of life.

Physical environment

The physical environment can mean a person's immediate surroundings, which may be their own home or that of others, such as a family home or residential care; it can also mean the public environment including shops, post office, banks, etc. and the wider environment, including air quality and other global factors. These aspects of the physical environment all have a role to play in people's psychological well-being, particularly if stress is experienced from the demands that the environment makes upon an individual relative to their ability to cope. This section will briefly discuss the first two meanings of 'physical environment.'

In Chapter 14 the meaning of 'home' is explored, with particular reference to psychological adjustments that older people may make when moving into residential care. The importance of home is considerable, in terms of the meanings embedded in a person's dwelling, their possessions, pets and clothing. Ninety-five per cent of people over the age of 60 years in the UK live in private households (OPCS 1993), although this drops to 76 per cent of people aged over 85. Home is good for people; in terms of psychological well-being, even being restricted to the home environment does not necessarily cause psychological problems. For example, in their survey of housebound older people, Lindsay and Thompson (1993) found no significant complaints of loneliness. Neither was there any significant increase in cases of depression, generalized anxiety and phobic disorders. Housebound respondents to Lindsay and Thompson's survey also remained in touch with people. They were in receipt of higher rates of contact with health and domiciliary services and of informal care from relatives, friends and neighbours.

With regard to the wider environment, an important issue is that of access to shops, transport services, public buildings and so on. For most older people this is not a problem, but for older people who have cognitive impairment, restricted mobility or sensory impairment there may be numerous obstacles to having access to the facilities and services outside the home that able people take for granted. This can result in a loss of independence, low morale and low self-esteem. These issues are relevant to people of any age who have impairments, and have been aptly described by Oliver (1983) as 'socially imposed restriction'.

Cognitive processes

Cognitive processes include functions such as memory, perception, attention and information processing. Although their functioning can be assessed independently, they are also interdependent and are affected by the other factors identified in Figure 7.1.

Memory

The complexity of memory highlights the intricacies of cognitive processes (see Figure 7.2). Although it is now generally agreed that there is some decline in memory as individuals age, this is not true for the different systems within the memory (Stuart-Hamilton 1994). In one formulation, memory can be seen as being composed of three stages: encoding, storage and retrieval of information (Atkinson et al 1996). In general, however, memory is identified as having two stages: short-term and long-term. Each has a number of components that are interconnected so that information can be used immediately, kept for a period then used, or stored for long periods then retrieved and used as necessary.

First, incoming messages from the sensory apparatus of sight, hearing, taste, smell, feeling/touch and a sense of position in space must be registered. This is important because, if any of these physical senses are defective, which is more likely as we grow older, messages will be received distorted or not at all. For example, visual changes, such as a loss of depth perception in older age, can cause misrepresentations being stored in the memory (Paton and Brown 1991).

Short-term memory can be divided into primary and working memory (Cohen 1996). Primary memory relates to information being held for a short time, then being either discarded, sent to working memory for manipulation and use, or sent for long-term storage. Ageing does not inherently result in a decrease in the capacity of primary memory, though some functions do decrease. Salthouse and Babcock (1991) found that as age increased, the number of digits that could be held in primary memory decreased, a decrement consistent with findings in other studies. However, Parkin and Walter (1991) found that, although

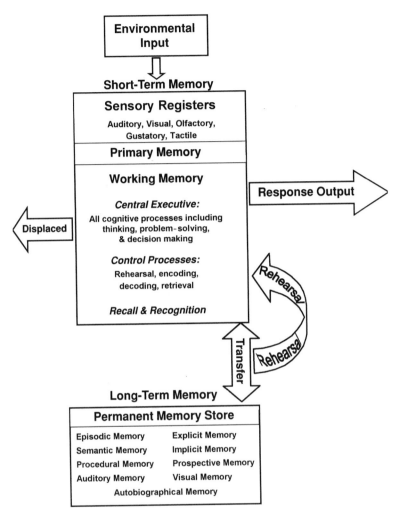

Figure 2: Model of Memory [adapted from Atkinson et al (1990; p289)]

Figure 7.2: Model of Memory. Adapted from Atkinson et al. (1990; p 289).

older subjects recall fewer items, there was no age decrement in their ability in recognition tasks or the rate at which they forgot information.

The working memory is where auditory and visual rehearsal occurs so that information can be remembered for longer periods. It also encodes and decodes information to aid storage and retrieval to and from the long-term memory (Cohen 1996). These functions take place under the control of a central executive (Logie 1999). Within this memory system, as people become older, there seems to be an overall reduction in functioning. For example, when a number of tasks requires simultaneous processing and/or storage for later use, older people perform badly (Wingfield et al 1988). Salthouse (1990), however, suggests this may be caused by slowed information-processing speed rather than memory deficits.

Long-term memory, or secondary memory, is identified as a store for information not held in the consciousness. Tulving (1985) divides it into three memory systems: episodic, semantic and procedural memory. Episodic memory relates to events and experiences that have had a personal impact on the individual, such as daily life events or as 'to-be-remembered' information. Cohen (1996) identifies a number of studies demonstrating a reduction with age in 'to-be-remembered' items. Semantic memory concerns language, facts, concepts and rules, while procedural memory relates to skills such as motor and cognitive skills. The decrements found with episodic memory are not always found with semantic or procedural memory (Cohen 1996). For example, in one semantic memory task studied, Light and Anderson (1983) found no significant differences between age groups in the ability to organize everyday activities, such as shopping. Procedural memory is now not seen as an independent system but part of implicit memory (Cohen 1996), which relates to memory not in conscious awareness. In a study by Howard and Howard (1992), it was suggested that implicit memory did not alter significantly with age. Another part of long-term memory is explicit memory, i.e. consciously recalling a recent event, and Howard and Howard (1992) found that older people were not as good at using explicit memory as younger people. However, some of these deficits may relate to encoding information for long-term storage. In a study by Hultsch and Dixon (1983), it was found that, if familiar material is being encoded, the deficit between old and young subjects is less than with novel material. One account of this is that older people may have difficulty inhibiting incoming irrelevant information (Hasher and Zacks 1988), thus altering the encoding process. Hamm and Hasher (1992) found that reduced response speeds in older subjects in rejecting irrelevant information in a comprehension test may relate to this encoding problem and could account for confusion shown by some older people when multiple information inputs occur simultaneously. Nonetheless, it is now generally accepted that older people have more difficulty retrieving information from long-term memory than younger people (Cohen 1996).

Although a number of deficits occur in various memory systems with old age, some of these can be compensated for by expertise and an increase in effort, concentration, attention and motivation. In a study by Cohen et al (1992) it was found that older university students received better coursework grades than younger students, but they did less well in examinations where timed recall and retrieval were required. They also found no age effect on remembering concepts, factual information or principles – a function of semantic memory.

Perception, attention and information processing

In order for information to be processed, it must be perceived. This involves a number of systems operating either at the same time or in a specified order. It also requires them to be functional. For example, alterations in the visual system of older people, such as difficulties in distinguishing facial patterns in reduced light or the auditory system resulting in hearing loss with high tones (Stuart-Hamilton 1994), can result in a distorted perception or a delay in accurate perception. In turn, this would result in inaccurate information being processed, or it taking a longer time to process this information. If sensory systems are in adequate functioning order, the information will be correctly perceived and processed.

A decline in sensory apparatus is not the only explanation for information being incorrectly processed. Another factor to consider is attention. It has been identified that older people are as able as younger people at sustaining attention (Salthouse 1982). However, it also seems that as people grow older they have difficulty selectively attending to information. Rabbitt (1979) found that older people were slower than younger people at a visual search task – one method to test selective attention. Similar results, i.e. reduced speed, were found when older people were required to divide attention between two tasks (Stuart-Hamilton 1994). Divided attention increases the complexity of a task, for example listening to the radio while trying to respond to someone's questions. The rationale given for this slowing is a confirmation of the age-times-complexity hypothesis in which reaction times are increased (i.e. a slower response rate) by an increase in age and/or the complexity of a task (Stuart-Hamilton 1994). However, although it has been demonstrated that older people process information more slowly than younger individuals, the differences become less and are more constant with practice (Rabbitt 1980). Also, Hasher and Zacks (1979) found that when a response becomes automatic there is only an insignificant difference between young and old. Another possible explanation is that since signal transmission in the nervous system slows with age (Stuart-Hamilton 1994), it may not be the actual processing of information but the physiological change that makes older people process information more slowly.

Individual differences

Two characteristics that differentiate individuals are their personalities and intellectual capacities. Although other attributes can be identified, these two are most often cited as changing in ways that clearly differentiate young and old. Thus, within this section of the model representing factors influencing individual psychological development (Figure 7.1), only these two elements will be examined.

Personality

In general, models of personality focus on either one trait at a time (single-trait theories) or a number of traits within the model (multi-trait theories). However, regardless of how personality structure is identified, some characteristics may change over time while others will not, but also the same attribute will change for some individuals but not for others (Atkinson et al 1996). It has also been proposed that there is a relatively stable core of personality characteristics. In a study by Schaie and Parham (1976) using subjects in the age bands of 21–28 years and 71–77 years, it was postulated that, once the personality core was formed, it did not change significantly over the life span.

Atkinson et al (1996) also suggest that environmental and cultural factors can influence some aspects of an individual's personality. This leads to an alternative view of personality development, identified as constructivist, which states that personality changes through a number of stages in an individual's life span (Hampson 1988). This could account for Erikson's (1964) position that not only do individuals change between different stages in the life span but also within a single stage. For example, in old age it may be possible to move from one end of the developmental conflict integrity vs. despair to the other (see pages 94–95 for definitions of integrity vs. despair). Thus, when taking a constructivist approach, it can be seen that, rather than personality becoming more rigid in old age, it is just as able to change and restructure to resolve developmental conflicts.

It is difficult to state which of these views is correct – stable personality or changeable one – as there is evidence to support both positions (Hampson 1988). These difficulties are compounded by the introduction of personality types for particular health problems, such as the 'C' personality, or cancer-prone personality, though evidence for this personality type is not conclusive (Taylor 1995). Taylor, however, notes that there is more evidence for a type 'A' personality, characterized by people who easily become aggressive, are impatient and competitive, and type 'B' personality, characterized by people who are less competitive, calmer and more introspective. In a study by Strube et al (1985), it was found that people with type A and type B personalities retain these into old age, making it more difficult for type As to adjust to reduced agility and decreased cognitive-processing speed associated with growing older.

Some aspects of personality, however, do seem to change in quality. For example, Eysenck (1987) found that neuroticism decreases with age and that older people are less prone to large mood swings. Also, as people get older, they become more introverted. Consequently, it is reasonable to assume that the ageing personality varies considerably between individuals, hence there is no 'typically old' personality (Stuart-Hamilton 1994). Also, personality seems to be formed at an early stage of development, with slight adjustments as people get older but with no radical changes unless physical/mental health, social or economic factors intervene.

Intellect

Intelligence is not an easy concept to define, with characteristics ranging from an ability to think abstractly to a global capacity to act purposefully and be able to solve specific problems (Curzon 1997). This variation fits the notion that intelligence is about not only academic ability, but also practical abilities (Atkinson et al 1996). It is because of this variation that age and intelligence have no simple relationship. However, some evidence does exist of an intellectual decline with age, though it is not global (Stuart-Hamilton 1994). Thus, the concept must be deconstructed to identify the extent to which age may have an effect.

Intelligence is now conventionally separated into fluid intelligence and crystallized intelligence (Horn and Cattell 1967). Fluid intelligence relates to an ability to solve problems where there is no previously known solution, either from an educational or cultural background. This generally shows a decline from the age of 60 years old and can intuitively be related to performance based upon psychomotor speed which declines with age (Stuart-Hamilton 1996). Crystallized intelligence includes items such as vocabulary and skills involving a high degree of pre-learned knowledge. It consists of information that has previously been fixed in the mind, i.e. 'crystallized'. A fairly consistent finding is that crystallized intelligence does not decline with age – and in some instances improves.

There are also a number of intervening variables that can aid intellectual functioning in older people. For example, Charness (1981) found that older chess players were as good as younger ones because of experience and the strategies they had developed over the years. Baltes and Willis (1982) demonstrate that training is able to improve task performance in older people. In a study by Gold et al (1995), it was shown that the intellectual abilities of older men completing a battery of psychological tests forty years after they were first taken were relatively stable. The changes noted in this study were an increase in vocabulary score, but a decrease in arithmetic scores, the ability to solve verbal analogies and non-verbal skills. These negative results were not easy to interpret because factors such as health, nutritional state, lifestyle, physical condition and life experiences could have affected the results.

This exemplifies how problematic it can be to compare young with old using intelligence tests. For example, because of psychomotor slowing, older people are disadvantaged at completing timed tests (Stuart-Hamilton 1996). Also, the average amount of education received by someone in their 20s now is much greater than for someone in their 20s 40–50 years ago. He suggested one way to control for these variables is by using a longitudinal design, but this would take 50–60 years to follow individuals from age 20 to age 70–80, being very expensive to run and likely to have a high drop-out rate. Thus, because of experimental difficulties, the findings of a general decline in intellectual abilities of old people are not very robust.

Relationships

Relationships are a fundamental part of our social structure. They meet a social need but are also required for survival. For example, an infant, of whatever species, needs contact with at least one other responsible individual to ensure biological survival. There also seems to be an innate capacity for children to respond in a complementary way to their carers - parents or others – to ensure this biologically important relationship is mutually satisfying (Durkin 1988). Thus, throughout our lives we develop reciprocating relationships with others to ensure biological, psychological and social survival.

There are a number of theoretical approaches to relationship development (Argyle 1988). A useful model is that of Levinger (1983), who postulates a linear pattern of acquaintance, build-up, consolidation, deterioration and ending. Argyle suggests that the elements of a relationship are activities, goals and conflicts, rules, skills, concepts and beliefs, and power and roles. How an older individual accommodates change in these factors can relate to a number of issues. In a study by Swan et al (1991), focusing on retirement, it was found that those who believed they were 'forced' to retire felt psychologically less healthy than those without such a belief. These results reflect difficulties some people had in accommodating to changes in most of the elements identified above. In contrast to this, Stuart-Hamilton (1994 p. 121) states, 'For the majority, retirement brings little change in satisfaction with life.' He further suggests that often the outcome of how many of these relationship changes are managed depends upon the individual's previous personality. It can also depend upon how the conflicts identified earlier in this chapter had been resolved (Erikson 1964). Thus it can be suggested that relationships will not automatically deteriorate in old age, though the influential factors as identified above will affect how they will be developed and maintained in old age.

It is important to note that an element of relationship development and maintenance is the emotional content of that relationship. Consequently, how this changes as an individual ages will affect the relationship. Although it is not clear what connection there is between emotions and ageing, emotions seem to become less extreme as people get older (Walton and Beck 1993). It has also been proposed that emotional capacity is well maintained in old age and has an important function in relation to memory, motivation and social judgement (Isaacowitz et al 2000). However, Jorm (2000) suggests that there may be a reduction in emotional responsiveness but an increase in emotional control with ageing. This could relate to changes in circumstances, such as physical health, environmental factors, social factors, family issues and financial issues – all of which can have an impact on an individual's emotional state. For example, it was found that financial loss equated to reduced self-worth and depression in older people (Krause et al 1991), which can have a detrimental effect on relationships. As with many of the areas of psychological development in older age already discussed, there is a mixed picture with deterioration not being an automatic response to ageing.

Social and financial factors

As identified above, social and financial factors have an effect on how older people feel about themselves and the environment in which they live. This is supported by Katona (1994), who suggests that, apart from the biological component, social factors, such as poverty, poor physical health and loneliness, play an important part in the development of depression in the older population. Scrutton (1989) suggests that a number of the difficulties experienced by older people in these areas are socially constructed, driven by myths which can often become reality. For example, Coleman (1999) cites a number of studies that have found that older people negatively stereotype themselves as being burdensome and unproductive.

Although all of the influencing factors identified thus far are linked, it can also be useful to examine them separately. Social issues, such as restrictions in mobility and social supports, have been identified as important factors in the development of mental health problems. Impairment, disability and handicap, which often result in social restrictions, have been found by Prince et al (1997) to result in depression. Social support has also been identified as an important factor in maintaining mental health. Oxman et al (1992), in a study of 1962 older people living in the community, found that there was a significant association between depression and social support (specifically instrumental in nature) and that an adequate amount of this form of support predicted a reduction in depression. These results seem to fit general expectations of psychological problems in older people. However, this is not always the case. For example, in a study of loneliness in people aged 75 years and older in London, it was found that, though those living alone tended to have more social services contact, their morbidity was no higher than in those living with others (Iliffe et al 1992).

It has already been identified that economic factors can affect the psychological well-being of older people (see Krause et al 1991). It has been well established that many older people have become financially disadvantaged once they retire (Walker 1990), which can affect psychological well-being because of the resultant economic and social restrictions. It is often assumed that older people who grew up during the Great Depression, when economic restrictions were common, would have learned to be resistant to these. In a study by Capsi and Elder (1986), this was shown not to be the case. They found that working-class women who grew up during the depression had lower ratings of self-esteem than middle-class women growing up during the same period. Socio-economic status may also have an effect on an individual's cognitive abilities. Brayne and Calloway (1990) studied whether socio-economic status may affect Mini Mental State Examination (MMSE) results when screening for dementia. They found that people grouped as manual workers as opposed to non-manual had lower MMSE scores, indicating more severe cognitive impairment. It was suggested, however, that these results needed further investigation as there is no clear cause-and-effect relationship. Thus, from the evidence presented above, it can be surmised that social and economic factors have an effect on the psychological well-being of older people.

Education

In order that learning be effective, a number of the psychological systems needs to be intact. However, expertise can overcome some deterioration in cognitive functioning in old age (Cohen 1996). As shown above, crystallized intelligence remains intact and only fluid intelligence shows a decline (Stuart-Hamilton 1996). It was also identified that not all aspects of fluid intelligence decline and that strategies previously learned can increase retention and the utilization of new material. Also, although information processing slows with age, information is still processed. Therefore, if an educational experience allows enough time, such as being assessed by essay rather than in a timed examination, learning can still take place and in some respects be more effective than with a younger person because of the larger pool of experience and knowledge. In a study by Haught et al (2000), it was found that the older age group was more confident than the younger one at problem-solving and, although taking longer to complete a concept-identification task, did not have significantly more errors than the younger group.

Memory is also required for learning. It was shown above that, although there is a general decrement in memory functioning, a number of areas remain intact or are reduced because of the effect of other systems. For example, it was stated that implicit memory does not seem to alter significantly with age. Sensory memory is likely to change because of deficits in sensory systems, such as hearing or vision. Consequently, this will affect information that reaches primary memory. If it is distorted, it will be incorrectly processed and remembered. Also, because recognition remains intact with older people, even though there is a decrease in the ability to recall, learning programmes that use visual aids are more likely to be effective.

Other areas identified in Figure 7.1, such as physical health, environmental, social and financial factors will also have an impact on an older person's educational motivation and ability. Thus, if poor nutrition, physical illness or social and financial constraints are being experienced, this can affect an individual's ability to learn. If, however, all of these barriers were removed and an adequate time was given, learning in old age would be able to take place. Also, if it were the case that older people were unable to learn, organizations such as the University of the Third Age would be unlikely to have sustained growth as it has since its inception in 1973 (http://www.u3ac.freeserve.co.uk/about.htm).

Culture and ethnicity

The population of the United Kingdom is diverse in terms of culture and ethnicity, and the proportion of older people from minority ethnic groups is rising as people reach retirement age (Warnes 1996).

It could be argued that there are potential problems facing older people from minority ethnic groups within the UK. As well as coping with the normal losses that can be associated with old age, such as the loss of health or the death of a partner, from ethnic minority groups older people may be coping with additional losses associated with migration from their homeland. These losses may be of status and role, the change of language or the loss of a familiar environment and contact with family and friends. Issues surrounding ethnicity are developed further in Chapter 11. Psychological well-being may be affected by encounters with cultural insensitivity and racial prejudice – and 'double jeopardy' may occur due to the double disadvantage of being both old and not white.

In practical terms, language barriers may cause difficulties for older people who require information or services but do not speak or read English or for whom English is not their first language. Sensory impairment can compound the language barrier, all resulting potentially in a loss of choice and involvement. This in turn can lead to powerlessness and a loss of self-esteem. Norman (1985) describes the isolation that can occur when a person is unable to gain access to treatment, support and care due to language, culture, skin colour or religious belief. When access to treatment is gained, there may be problems in obtaining culturally sensitive assessments, particularly with regard to the assessment of cognitive function. For example, some bedside tests are culturally biased, asking questions such as the date of World War I or the name of the Prime Minister. These types of questions may not be answered correctly by a person who is unfamiliar with British history and culture.

Conclusion

This chapter has aimed to clarify the relationships between a variety of psychological factors in ageing. It used a model that has a bio-psycho-social framework (Figure 7.1). It also identified that many psychological processes remain intact into old age, with some even improving. However, because of the strong interplay between different psychological components, if there is a deficit in one area it will inevitably affect the others. It has been highlighted that, when caring for an older person, it is important not to assume psychological deficits but to recognize that their previous physical condition, experiences, cultural development and knowledge have an effect on their current presentation and also that more time is needed for processing and responding to different situations, especially if they are complex. Finally, it is necessary to recognize that, when caring for an older person, this can be affected by not only our negative attitudes towards ageing but also their own negative attitudes towards themselves. In conclusion, those caring for older people must recognize their adult status and that psychological deficits are more likely to be the result of illness, either psychological or physical and not an inevitable consequence of ageing.

References

Argyle M (1988) Social Relationships. In: Hewstone M, Stroebe W, Codol J-P and Stephenson G M (eds) Introduction to Social Psychology pp. 222–245. Oxford: Blackwell.

Atkinson R L, Atkinson R C, Smith E E, Bem D J and Hildegard E R (1990) Introduction to Psychology 10th edn. New York: Harcourt Brace Jovanovich.

Atkinson R L, Atkinson R C, Smith E E, Bem D J and Nolen-Hoeksema S (1996) Hildegard's Introduction to Psychology 12th edn. New York: Harcourt Brace Jovanovich.

Baltes P and Willis S L (1982) Plasticity and enhancement of intellectual functioning in old age. In: Craik F M and Trehub A S (eds) Aging and Cognitive Processes pp. 353–389. New York: Plenum.

Bolla K I, Lindgren K N, Bonaccorsy C and Bleecker M L (1991) Memory Complaints in Older Adults – fact or fiction? Archives of Neurology 48 (1): 61–64.

Brayne C and Calloway P (1990) The Association of Education and Socioeconomic Status with the Mini Mental State Examination and the Clinical Diagnosis of Dementia in Elderly People. Age and Ageing 19 (2): 91–96.

Capsi A and Elder GH (1986) Life satisfaction in old age: linking social psychology and history. Journal of Psychology and Aging 1 (1): 18–26.

Charness N (1981) Aging and skilled problem solving. Journal of Experimental Psychology: General 110 (1): 21–38.

Cohen G, Stanhope N and Conway M A (1992) Age differences in the retention of knowledge by young and elderly students. British Journal of Developmental Psychology 10 (2): 153–164.

Cohen G (1996) Memory and Learning in Normal Ageing. In: Woods R T (ed) Handbook of the Clinical Psychology of Ageing pp. 43–58. Chichester: John Wiley and Sons.

Coleman P (1993) Psychological Ageing. In: Bond J, Coleman P and Peace S (eds) Ageing in Society pp. 62–88. London: Sage.

Coleman P G (1999) Identity Management in Later Life. In: Woods R T (ed) Psychological Problems of Ageing pp. 49–72. Chichester: John Wiley and Sons, Ltd.

Cumming E and Henry W (1961) Growing Old: the Process of Disengagement. New York: Basic Books.

Curzon L B (1997) Teaching in Further Education 5th edn. London: Cassell.

Durkin K (1988) The Social Nature of Social Development. In: Hewstone M, Stroebe W, Codol J-P and Stephenson G M (eds) Introduction to Social Psychology pp. 39–59. Oxford: Blackwell.

Erikson E H (1964) Insight and Responsibility. London: Faber.

Eysenck H J (1987) Personality and Ageing: an Exploratory Analysis. Journal of Social Behaviour and Personality 3 (1): 11–21.

Flicker C, Ferris S H and Reisberg B (1993) A longitudinal Study of Cognitive Function in Elderly Persons with Subjective Memory Complaints. Journal of the American Geriatrics Society 41 (10): 1029–1032.

Gold D P, Andres D, Etezadi J and Arbuckle T (1995) Structural equation model of intellectual change and continuity and predictors of intelligence in older men. Psychology and Aging 10 (2): 294–303.

Grant I, Heaton R K, McSweeny A J, Adams K M and Timms R M (1982) Neuropsychological findings in hypoxemic chronic obstructive pulmonary disease. Archives of Internal Medicine 142 (8): 1470–1476.

Grundy E, Bowling A and Farqhar M (1997) Living Well into Old Age. London: Age Concern England/Joseph Rowntree Foundation findings.

Hamm V P and Hasher L (1992) Age and availability of inferences. Psychology and Aging 7 (1): 56–64.

Hampson S E (1988) The Construction of Personality 2nd edn. London: Routledge.

Hasher L and Zacks R T (1988) Working memory, comprehension and aging: a review and a new view. In: Bower G H (ed) The Psychology of Learning and Motivation pp. 193–225. New York: Academic Press.

Hasher L and Zacks R T (1979) Automatic and effortful processes in memory. Journal of Experimental Psychology: General 108: 356–388.

Haught P A, Hill L A, Nardi A H and Walls R T (2000) Perceived ability and level of education as predictors of traditional and practical adult problem solving. Experimental Aging Research 26 (1): 89–101.

Havighurst R J (1963) Successful ageing. In: Williams R H, Tibbitts C and Donahue W (eds) Processes of Ageing volume 1 pp. 299–320. New York: Athergon.

Holland C A and Rabbitt R (1991) The course and causes of cognitive change with advancing age. Reviews in Clinical Gerontology 1: 79–94.

Horn J L and Cattell R B (1967) Age differences in fluid and crystallised intelligence. Acta Psychologia 26 (2): 107–129.

Howard D and Howard J H (1992) Adult age differences in the rate of learning serial patterns: evidence from direct and indirect tests. Psychology and Aging 7: 232–241.

Hultsch D F and Dixon R A (1983) The role of pre-experimental knowledge in text processing in adulthood. Experimental Aging Research 9 (1): 7–22.

Iliffe S, Tai S S, Haines A, Gallivan S, Goldenberg E, Booroff A and Morgan P (1992) Are elderly people living alone an at risk group? British Medical Journal 305 (6860): 1001–1004.

Isaacowitz D M, Charles S T and Carstensen L L (2000) Emotion and cognition. In: Craik F I M and Salthouse T A (eds) The Handbook of Aging and Cognition 2nd edn. pp. 539–631. Mahwah, New Jersey: Lawrence Erlbaum Associates.

Jorm A F I (2000) Does old age reduce risks of anxiety and depression? A review of epidemiological studies across the life span. Psychological Medicine 30 (1): 11–22.

Katona C L E (1994) Approaches to the Management of Depression in Old Age. Gerontology 40 (supplement 1): 5–9.

Krause N, Jay G and Liang J (1991) Financial strain and psychological well-being among American and Japanese elderly. Psychology and Aging 6 (2): 170–181.

Laslett P (1989) A Fresh Map of Life: The Emergence of the Third Age. London: Weidenfeld and Nicholson.

Levinger G (1983) Development and change. In: Kelley H H (ed) Close Relationships. New York: Freeman.

Levinson D J (1980) Toward a conception of the adult life course. In: Smelser N J and Erikson E H (eds) Themes of Work and Love in Adulthood. London: Grant McIntyre.

Light L L and Anderson P A (1983) Memory for scripts in young and older adults. Memory and Cognition 11 (5): 435–444.

Lindsay J and Thompson C (1993) Housebound elderly people: definition, prevalence and characteristics. International Journal of Geriatric Psychiatry 8: 231–237.

Logie R H (1999) Working memory. The Psychologist 12 (4): 174–178.

McGlone J, Gupta S, Humphrey D, Oppenheimer S, Mirsen T and Evans D R (1990) Screening for Early Dementia Using Memory Complaints From Patients and Relatives. Archives of Neurology 47 (11): 1189–1193.

Norman A (1985) Triple Jeopardy: growing old in a second homeland. London: Centre for Policy on Ageing.

Office of Population Censuses and Surveys (OPCS) (1993) The 1991 Census Persons Aged 60 and Over in Great Britain. London: HMSO.

Oliver (1983) Social Work with Disabled People. London: Macmillan.

Oxman T E, Berkman L F, Kasl S, Freeman D H Jr and Barrett J (1992) Social Support and Depressive Symptoms in the Elderly. American Journal of Epidemiology 135 (4): 356–368.

Parkin A J and Walter B M (1991) Aging, short term memory and frontal dysfunction. Psychobiology 19: 175–179.

Paton D and Brown R (1991) Lifespan Health Psychology: Nursing Problems and Interventions: 198–227. London: Harper Collins.

Prince M J, Harwood R H, Blizard R A and Mann A H (1997) Impairment, disability and handicap as risk factors for depression in old age. The Gospel Oak Project V. Psychological Medicine 27 (2): 311–321.

Rabbitt P M A (1979) Some experiments and a model for changes in attentional selectivity with old age. In: Hoffmeister F and Muller C (eds) Bayer Symposium VII. Evaluation of Change. Bonn: Springer.

Rabbitt P M A (1980) A fresh look at reaction times in old age. In: Stein D G (ed) The Psychobiology of Aging: Problems and Perspectives. New York: Elsevier.

Rabbitt P and Abson V (1990) 'Lost and found': some logical and methodological limitations of self-report questionnaires as tools to study cognitive ageing. British Journal of Psychology 81 (1): 1–16.

Salthouse T (1982) Adult Cognition. New York: Springer.

Salthouse T A (1990) Working memory as a processing resource in cognitive aging: limited resource models of cognitive development. Developmental Review 10: 101–124.

Salthouse T A and Babcock R L (1991) Decomposing adult age differences in working memory. Developmental Psychology 27: 763–776.

Schaie K W (1990) Optimization of cognitive functioning. In: Baltes P M and Baltes M M (eds) Successful Aging: perspectives from the behavioural sciences pp. 94–117. Cambridge (Mass): Cambridge University Press.

Schaie K W and Parham A (1976) Stability of adult personality traits: fact or fable? Journal of Personality and Social Psychology 34: 146–158.

Scrutton S (1989) Counselling Older People. London: Edward Arnold.

Sherwin B B (1997) Estrogen effects on cognition in menopausal women. Neurology 48 (supplement 7): S21–S26.

Strube M J, Berry J M, Goza B K and Fennimore D (1985) Type A behaviour, age and psychological well-being. Journal of Personality and Social Psychology 49 (1): 203–218.

Stuart-Hamilton I (1994) The Psychology of Ageing 2nd edn. London: Jessica Kingsley Publishers.

Stuart-Hamilton I (1996) Intellectual Changes in Late Life. In: Woods R T (ed) Handbook of the Clinical Psychology of Ageing pp. 23–41. Chichester: John Wiley and Sons.

Swan G E, Dame A and Carmelli D (1991) Involuntary retirement, Type A behaviour, and current functioning in elderly men: 27-year follow-up of the Western Collaborative Group Study. Psychology and Aging 6 (3): 384–391.

Taylor S E (1995) Health Psychology 3rd edn. New York: McGraw-Hill, Inc.

Tulving E (1985) How many memory systems are there? American Psychologist 40: 385–398.

Walker A (1990) The Benefits of Old Age? In: McEwen E (ed) Age: The Unrecognised Discrimination pp. 58–70. London: Age Concern.

Walton C G and Beck C K (1993) The Aged Adult. In: Rawlins R D, Williams S R and Beck C K (eds) Mental Health – Psychiatric Nursing – A holistic life-cycle approach pp. 801–824. St. Louis: Mosby.

Warnes T (1996) The age structure and ageing of the ethnic groups. In: D Coleman and J Salt (eds) Ethnicity in the 1991 Census, Volume One: demographic characteristics of the ethnic minority population pp. 151–177. London: OPCS.

Wilkie F and Eisdorfer C (1971) Intelligence and blood pressure in the aged. Science 172 (986): 959–963.

Wingfield A, Stine E A L, Lahar C J and Aberdeen J S (1988) Does the capacity of working memory change with age? Experimental Aging Research 16 (2/3): 73–77.

Young M and Schuller T (1983) The New Prospects for Retirement. In: Johnson J and Slater S (eds) Ageing and Later life. London: Sage.

CHAPTER 8

Abnormal psychology in old age

NICKY HAYES AND HENRY A MINARDI

Introduction

Normal psychological development in old age is examined in the previous chapter. The discussion evolved from a model identifying factors that contribute to normal psychological development: a context of individual, biological, social, cultural and environment influences. This highlights the complexity of the process of growing older, any part of which, if adversely affected, may lead to abnormal changes. It is the purpose of this chapter to explore some of the influences that may lead to abnormal psychological development in old age and then to describe the effects of abnormal development in terms of mental health problems. The identification and description of mental health problems in themselves would be insufficient for an understanding of abnormal psychology without considering the impact of these problems on the individual and upon their informal carers. These will, therefore, be discussed, with an emphasis upon the range of effects that these problems may create for carers. It should be noted that while there is a number of available treatments and interventions, such as medication and psychotherapy, there is insufficient space to discuss these in this chapter though references to help the reader obtain information from other sources will be given.

Three interacting components of abnormal psychology in old age are summarized in Figure 8.1. The first element is that of the *influences* that may cause abnormal psychological development, second is the *effects* of abnormal development as manifested in mental health problems, and third is the *care and treatment* of problems that occur. Underlying each component is the interaction between biological, psychological and social factors within which reside the thoughts, feelings and behaviours of individuals. The influences and effects of abnormal psychological devel-

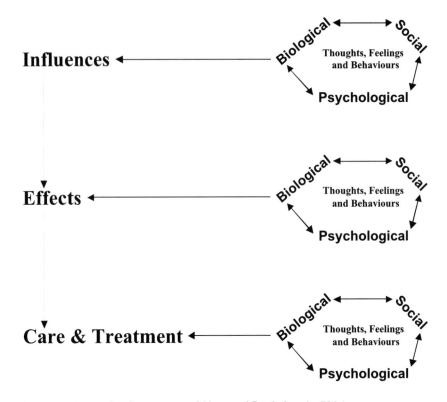

Figure 8.1: Interacting Components of Abnormal Psychology in Old Age

opment will be discussed later. First the prevalence of mental health problems in old age will be identified.

Prevalence of mental health problems in old age

The Office of Population Censuses and Surveys (OPCS 1993) has identified a general increase in the ageing population. Consequently there is
more likely to be a proportionate increase in the number of people over 65
years old who may develop mental health problems and their attendant
care implications.

It is important to differentiate between the care required by individuals
who develop mental health problems in old age and those who have grown
older with an established mental health problem. Community prevalence
studies of older people and mental health have found that depression is the
most common problem, followed by dementia, while other mental health
problems are between 0% and 1.1% (Kirby et al, 1997, Lawlor et al 1994,
Lobo et al 1995, Saunders et al 1993, see Table 8.1). All of these studies use

Table 8.1: Prevalence of Diagnostic Cases

Diagnosis	Ramsay et al (1991)	Walker et al (1995)	Saunders et al (1993)	Lawlor et al (1994)	Lobo et al (1995)	Kirby et al (1997)
Organic/Dementia	61%	16%	4.7%	5.5%	5.5%	4.1%
Depression	10%	27%	10%	13.1%	4.8%	10.3%
Anxiety	not assessed	not assessed	0.9%	1.1%	0.6%	0.8%
Phobia	not assessed	not assessed	0.8%	0.0%	not assessed	0.2%
Hypochondriasis	not assessed	not assessed	0.8%	not assessed	not assessed	0.0%
Obsessional	not assessed	not assessed	0.1%	0.0%	not assessed	0.0%
Schizophrenia	not assessed	not assessed	0.2%	0.0%	see other	0.0%
Other	N/A	N/A	N/A	N/A	0.9%*	N/A

*(Schizophrenia, Paranoid delusions, Alcoholism and Delirium)

Study sample details

1. Kirby et al (1997); Interview t = 1232; GMS-AGECAT; 1991 Dublin Census.
2. Lawlor et al (1994); Interview t = 451; GMS-AGECAT; one GP group practice.
3. Lobo et al (1995); Interview t = 1080; DSM-III-R; Zaragoza Municipal Census List; Other: Schizophrenia, Paranoid delusions, Alcoholism and Delirium.
4. Ramsay et al (1991); Interview t = 119; Mini-Mental State Exam (MMSE), Geriatric Depression Schedule (GDS), General Health Questionnaire (GHQ-30), BAS of the short CARE; Acute Elderly Medical Admission units in 2 General Hospitals; + 29% of patients interviewed, though not diagnosed as depressed, had significant symptoms.
5. Saunders et al (1993), Interview t = 5222; GMS-AGECAT; Liverpool Family Practitioner Committee list of GP patients; Other: not specified.
6. Walker et al (1995); Interview t = 109; Brief Assessment Schedule (BAS) of the short CARE; General Hospital Accident & Emergency Department.

the standardized research tool, GMS-AGECAT (Geriatric Mental State Automated Geriatric Examination for Computer-Assisted Taxonomy – Copeland et al 1986). However, what appears to be the case, and is shown in Table 8.1, is that these is a difference in the amount of depression and dementia found between in-patient units in a general hospital (Ramsay et al 1991), an Accident and Emergency Department (Walker et al 1995) and the general population (Kirby et al 1997, Lawlor et al 1994, Lobo et al 1995, Saunders et al 1993). What this identifies is that depression is more likely to be found in the general population, while it is more likely that there will be high levels of dementia on in-patient units in general hospitals.

Psychological disturbances with older people

All of the mental health problems identified in Table 8.1 can affect both young and older adults. Also, the manifestation of these problems may be similar in both the young and old, though differences can also be identified. For example, Cohen et al (1999) suggest that symptoms of mania are the same in both age groups, although there are longer periods of remission with older adults. Schaub and Linden (2000) contend that there is not a significant difference in the way anxiety is manifested between young and old but that these disorders decrease with age; however, gender differences remain, with more women than men having an anxiety disorder. This section will now examine what may influence the development of these disorders in older people and how they may manifest themselves.

Bio-psycho-social influences

Biological influences

Mental health problems in old age may have a biological basis that arises from general physical health or from direct brain pathology. The effect that physical health, including cardiovascular and respiratory function, can have on psychological well-being has been outlined in Chapter 7. This section will briefly discuss the biological basis of mental health problems in old age. The cognitive and behavioural features of disorders will be described in more detail later in this chapter.

Mental health problems tend to be described within psychiatry as either *functional* or *organic*. Depression is the major *functional* disorder of old age, while dementia and delirium are the main *organic* disorders. As described in psychiatric terms, the latter type of disorders arise from pathology, that is from some form of brain malfunction. This division into functional and organic is possibly misleading in that there is some evidence that depression may also have biological origins. For example, depression occurs frequently after a cerebrovascular accident, in which context it is now considered to be a response to brain injury rather than a simple psychological reaction to physical disability (Primeau 1988). In other cases, it can still be argued that to dismiss depression purely as an 'affective' or mood disorder arising from loneliness or bereavement in old age is an obstacle to its recognition and treatment (Pitt 1997). In terms of overall physical health, factors that may lead to or contribute to depression also include sensory impairment, pain, hypothyroidism and poor general health.

Although dementia in old age used to be known as 'senile dementia', it is now recognized that in many cases the underlying psychopathology is the same as for the Alzheimer-type dementia – a term previously used for 'pre-senile' dementia. The pathology of Alzheimer's is characterized by the formation of structures known as *plaques* within the brain and *neurofibrillary tangles* within neurones. The causes and processes involved in the disease are not fully understood, although there is known to be a genetic contribution in some cases (Fitch 1988, Antuono and Beyer 1999). Risk factors include smoking, hypertension and atherosclerosis (Prince 1995), though evidence is inconclusive and requires further research. Also, although aluminium exposure has been found to be associated with Alzheimer's in some studies, Doll's (1993) review concludes that confounding variables may have been the cause of a positive association. In other words, the review's findings suggested that there was not enough causal evidence between aluminium exposure and Alzheimer's.

Psychological influences

Mental health problems in old age may be influenced by psychological factors, such as the person's personality type, past behaviours and coping mechanisms. It has already been noted that the data on prevalence of mental health problems depend upon the assessment methods and diagnostic criteria used, which can be complex and within which people do not always fit. To exemplify this complexity, Pitt (1996) lists obsessive personality as a predisposing factor for depression but also includes family and previous history of depression, loss of the mother at an early age and marital strife.

Social and ethnic influences

Many of the negative stereotypes of old age are tied in with the image of 'senility' – loss of mental faculties, dependency, incoherence and drooling. The image is of a non-person, whose identity and humanity can no longer be perceived. Featherstone and Hepworth (1993 p. 313) suggest that: 'In this prevailing imagery the afflicted individual has lost his or her power of self-control: of being able to express the self-identity that he or she believes others have come to expect.'

The image of senility is that of irreversible decline and powerlessness. There are profound implications for the way that stereotypical views may affect the way that older people who have mental health problems, such as dementia, are perceived and treated. For example, the process of being labelled and consequently treated as a dependent or worthless person is part of the 'malignant social psychology' described by Kitwood (1990) that leads to a loss of personhood, institutionalization and further dependency.

Deteriorating mental health still carries a stigma for some people, who may be reluctant to seek help because of a fear of being labelled as 'senile'; people who were born in the early twentieth century may also remember institutions such as the workhouse, and this may reinforce their reservations.

Some of the factors that may affect the psychological development of people from minority ethnic groups are outlined in Chapter 7. It is difficult to deduce the prevalence of mental health problems amongst older people from minority ethnic groups in the UK, owing to a lack of statistical data on ethnicity and the pattern of mental disorders and service use in all age groups. For example, Abas (1997) cites Cochrane and Bal (1989) who found that for all diagnoses, except schizophrenia, the rates of admissions to mental hospitals were lower among adults from minority ethnic groups than for people who were born in England. This does not necessarily mean that there is a lower rate of psychological disorders, such as depression, among people from minority ethnic groups, just that it may not be diagnosed, or services may not be being used by people from these groups.

Bio-psycho-social effects

While it can be argued that labelling an individual's mental or physical health problems can stigmatize them, resulting in a detrimental effect on their personal and social identity, it can also be beneficial to correctly identify a mental health problem to ensure appropriate care is given. For example, recognizing that memory loss may be caused by depression and not only by dementia can result in the appropriate care and treatment of the individual's depression. Thus, mental health problems and how they affect older people will be identified below.

Depression

This is the most common mental health problem identified in older people (see Table 8.1). However, it is not an inevitable consequence of ageing (Copeland et al 1999) or untreatable (Copeland 1999). The American Psychiatric Association (APA) in their Diagnostic and Statistical Manual of Mental Disorders, 4th edn. (DSM-IV), have categorized depression into major depressive disorder and dysthymic disorder – a less severe form of depression (APA 1994). Generally, there are no substantial differences in presenting symptoms between old and young people (Keogh and Roche 1996), though some may be more pronounced, such as physical problems, while others may not be present, such as feelings of guilt (Katona 1994). See Box 8.1 for a list of signs and symptoms of depression in older people.

With older people, when the severity of depression increases, there tends to be an increase in somatic complaints, such as constipation, psychomotor agitation/retardation, sleep disturbances of initial insomnia or late insomnia, frequently waking, a loss of libido and a loss of appetite (Blazer 1993). In some instances, there could also be biological mechanisms that precipitate a depressive episode, such as thyroid disease (Kivelä et al 1996). When physical illness is co-morbid with depression, it is thought there will be a less favourable outcome (Blazer 1993).

Poor physical health and disability have a strong association with depression, a finding that has been replicated on numerous occasions (Beekman et al 1995, Kivelä et al 1996, Prince et al 1997). Kennedy et al (1990), however, found that the acuteness rather than the severity or chronicity of a disability was more predictive of depression. Prince et al (1997) are cautious in their interpretations, and have difficulty in deciding whether impairment results in depression, or the other way around.

Psychological manifestations of depression are identified by the first twelve symptoms in Box 8.1, which describe how people feel about themselves. According to Keogh and Roche (1996), although there is not a substantial difference in presenting symptoms between the old and the young, some clinical features are more likely to occur in older people. Older people may experience an exaggeration of personal helplessness, are more likely to present with somatic complaints, are less likely to report psychological discomfort as depression, are less likely to feel guilty or worthless and may have delusions (Brodaty et al 1991, Blazer 1993,

---

Box 8.1: Depressive Signs and Symptoms (adapted from Blazer 1993)

Depressed mood
Sense of emptiness
Exaggeration of personal helplessness
Feelings of worthlessness
Withdrawal from social activities leading to boredom and loneliness
Anxiety
Distorted and unrealistic thoughts about self and social environment
Unwarranted pessimism about the future
Ruminations about past and present problems
Difficulty in concentrating
Memory loss
Thoughts of death or suicide
Insomnia, but sometimes hypersomnia
Psychomotor agitation and retardation
Older people are less likely to identify feelings of guilt or worthlessness
Older people are less likely to report psychological discomfort as
depression
Constipation
Weight loss
In older people, somatic symptoms (identified below) increase in
severity and frequency with increased severity of depression:

1. sleep problems
2. fatigue
3. dizziness
4. appetite changes
5. gastrointestinal symptoms

Katona 1994). Blazer (1993) also suggests that a lower satisfaction with life is associated with depression in older people. Tijhuis et al (1999) suggest that changes in mood and an increase in depression have been associated with loneliness, and have noted that an increase in loneliness is more likely to occur in people over 79 years of age. It is important to recognize that, with pessimistic thinking, thoughts of death and suicide are also likely to be present. These need to be taken seriously and appropriate questions asked in an attempt to detect suicidal intent. Box 8.2 outlines some possible questions that might help to identify such intent.

Many of the symptoms of depression can precipitate a reduction in social contact because of withdrawal from social activities and the rejection of others. Palsson and Skoog (1997) identify social deprivation, loneliness and poor quality of life as significant consequences of depression. With a reduction in the number of social contacts, there will be a reduction in support. This is an unfortunate dilemma because a decrease in social support can be a consequence of depression, yet adequate support is needed to reduce or prevent depression (Prince et al 1997).

Dementia

This is a disturbance of multiple-cognitive abilities that must include memory loss and deficits in a central-processing ability, such as problem-solving, language production and recognition, object recognition, and intellectual functioning (APA 1994). It is recognized as a syndrome in which

---

Box 8.2: Assessing Suicide Risk

Do you still get pleasure out of life?
Do you feel hopeful from day to day? / Do you think things will turn out well?
Are you able to face each day? / Do you ever wish not to wake up?
Do you feel life is a burden? / Do you wish to end it all?
Have you ever thought of ending your life? / At the moment, is there anything to live for?
Are you able to resist the thought?
Have you thought about the method of suicide?
Have you ever tried anything?
How likely are you to kill yourself?
Is there anything that might make you feel worse?

Look and listen for Suicide Trajectory warning signs: depressed mood, clearing affairs, dropping out/withdrawal, verbal threats, self-injurious behaviour.

Aquilina and Warner (1996) p. 33

---

the impairments identified above are the result of a global deterioration in cognitive functioning and memory (Cervilla et al 1997). Its prevalence in community-dwelling older people is from 4.1% in people over 65 years of age (Kirby et al 1997) to about 20% in those over the age of 80 (Woods 1999a). This, of course, means that 95% of people over 65 and 80% of people over 80 do not have dementia, demonstrating that it is not an inevitable part of the ageing process. Although there a number of types of dementia, this chapter will be referring to only three of these: Alzheimer's, vascular dementia and dementia with Lewy bodies. Other dementias are Pick's disease, dementias due to HIV infection, from head injury, Parkinson's disease, Huntington's disease, Creutzfeldt-Jakob disease (CJD) and substance-induced dementia.

For the diagnosis of Alzheimer's, there must be memory loss and at least one of the central-processing deficits of *aphasia* (language disturbance), *apraxia* (impaired ability to carry out motor activities despite intact motor function), *agnosia* (failure to recognize or identify objects despite intact sensory function) and a disturbance in executive functioning (i.e. planning, organizing, sequencing, abstracting) (APA 1994). Other central nervous system problems, substance misuse or systemic problems must be eliminated. Also, that the cognitive deficits cause significant impairment in social or occupational functioning and represent a significant decline from previous functional abilities must be recognized. The course is characterized by the gradual onset and a continuous, linear cognitive decline. It is now acknowledged that Alzheimer's is the most common form of dementia (Antuono and Beyer 1999), with mortality occurring 8-10 years after the manifestation of symptoms (APA 1994).

Vascular dementia displays similar signs and symptoms as Alzheimer's, with added focal neurological signs and evidence of cerebrovascular disease (APA 1994). Its course is described as a 'stepwise' deterioration, i.e., when a mini-cerebrovascular accident (mini-CVA) occurs that is insufficient to cause significant motor deficits, there will be a small deterioration in cognitive functioning. This will remain static until the next mini-CVA. The progress is variable and patchy with some areas of the brain not being affected (APA 1994).

A central feature in dementia with Lewy bodies is that there is a progressive cognitive decline of sufficient magnitude to interfere with normal social or occupational function (McKeith 1997). Memory impairment may not be present early in the illness but is present as it progresses.

McKeith also suggests that there is usually a fluctuating cognition, with pronounced variations in attention and alertness, and recurrent visual hallucinations that are well defined and detailed. Ballard et al (1998) have found that in both post-mortem and clinical studies 10%–20% of all cases of dementia are dementia with Lewy bodies.

The memory impairment caused by all of these dementias results in many physical problems. Examples of this can be seen in the various dangers relating to electric heaters or forgetting that the cooker is on, with the attendant possibility of fire. There is the possibility of going outside in inappropriate clothing for the time of year, which can cause physical illness. Eating and drinking inappropriately or forgetting to do so at all could cause physical problems. Also, because of perceptual misinterpretations, individuals may refuse help when in distress or be unable to understand situations and people that could be either physically dangerous or helpful. Orrell et al (2000) found that people with dementia who have poor physical health and have higher levels of dependency than others with dementia have a lower survival rate. Just as serious is the risk of taking an inadvertent overdose of medication because it has been forgotten that a dose had just been taken.

In the initial stages, a person with dementia may not have a reduction in social contacts as memory deficits will be patchy and covered up by making a joke of forgetfulness, putting the memory loss down to 'old age', or suggestions that this is how they have always been. As the dementia progresses, it becomes more difficult to use these strategies and memory lapses become more frequent. Recognizing this progression makes it more important to acknowledge Kitwood's (1993) premiss that there is a need to understand the whole of the person with dementia, not just their brain pathology. He suggests that an examination of the individual's personality, biography and social psychology is required to understand how dementia has developed and how it affects the individual sufferer and their 'significant others'. This acknowledges the importance of recognizing the impact of difficult life events, such as retirement, bereavement, physical illness or stressful conflicts, in shaping the progress of dementia (Adams 1996). Because of the symptoms of dementia, social supports are likely to be reduced or even rejected, which can place the individual at a disadvantage. For example, Orrell et al (2000) found a significant relationship between aspects of social support, such as receiving meals on wheels, having supportive relatives and attending a day centre, and an increase in the survival rate of people with dementia.

Acute confusional state

This is a clouded state of consciousness identified by a difficulty in concentrating, focusing attention and maintaining a direct and coherent train of thought (APA 1994). There are often perceptual disturbances, such as mistaking unfamiliar for familiar, and hallucinations and illusions – particularly visual and mixed visual-auditory hallucinations. Signs and symptoms are usually worse at night and with increased sleeplessness. Its course is such that it develops quickly over hours or days. If the cause is identified, e.g. infection, it can usually be effectively treated.

An acute confusional state (delirium) can be caused by a single biological disorder or disease, or it can be multi-factorial (Byrne 1997). Thus cardiovascular disorders, respiratory infection or urinary-tract infection can cause delirium. It is also possible that delirium could be superimposed on to an already existing cognitive deficit, such as Alzheimer's, by the presence of incontinence, constipation, sensory deficits, environmental change or drug treatments (Byrne 1997). People in an acute confusional state tend to misperceive external stimuli, such as a sound being heard as louder than it actually is. Often there are visual hallucinations, which can be frightening and cause distress. Because of disruptive behaviour, such as aggression or responding to hallucinations, social contact becomes difficult with a person who is in an acute confusional state. This is made more problematic because they will lack the expected social reciprocity, that is being able to return appropriate social responses.

Anxiety

The American Psychiatric Association (1994) has identified a number of features that must be present for the person to be identified as having an anxiety disorder. There must be excessive anxiety and worry for the past six months about activities/events relating to at least three of the following: restlessness/feeling on edge, easily fatigued, concentration difficulties, irritability, muscular tension and sleep disturbance. Other symptoms may be present, such as trembling, shaking, shortness of breath, palpitations, sweating, dry mouth, dizziness, nausea, diarrhoea and flushes or chills and, also, that the anxiety is not secondary to another disorder, and that it does not occur only during mood disturbance. It exists in the absence of any physical disorder and can have a deleterious effect on social and occupational functioning. It is also common to find anxiety associated with depression in older people.

Phobia

Although a separate disorder from anxiety, the American Psychiatric Association (1994) categorizes phobic illnesses as part of the umbrella heading 'Anxiety'. Phobias present with similar symptoms to those of anxiety states described above, but relate to particular situations. Avoidance of the situation, object or event is a key characteristic. Also included within criteria for phobias are panic attacks that are identified by discrete periods of severe fear in which four or more of the anxiety symptoms identified above are present (APA 1994).

In older people the most common phobias are fear of animals or heights and there is nearly a 2:1 prevalence ratio of women to men (Krasucki et al 1998). With social phobias, there is a significant and constant fear of situations that have a social or performance function (APA 1994). Exposure to these situations causes severe anxiety and may even result in a panic attack. Major depression has been significantly linked to social phobias, and, if a person presents with major depression, a co-existing social phobia needs to be ruled out (Stein et al 1999).

With anxiety and phobias, biological effects relate to the symptoms experienced, such as palpitations, sweating, trembling, dry mouth and pupil dilation. There is often an inability to go out or confront the feared object or situation, with a resultant avoidance. However, it was found that women with phobias were more likely to comply with a screening routine for breast cancer than those without a phobia (Desai et al 1999). Chronic physical disability due to conditions such as arthritis and sensory impairment are associated with high rates of subjective anxiety and avoidance (Lindesay 1997). He also notes that older people sometimes develop what seems to be an excessive fear of falling when there are no physical supports visible. However, there is some evidence that this is associated with a disturbance in the vestibulo-ocular and righting reflexes (Lindesay 1997). Generally, there is a tendency for older people to somatize, thus blaming physical causes for their highly aroused emotional state (Fuentes and Cox 1997).

Schizophrenia

Individuals with schizophrenia commonly present with symptoms relating to distorted thinking of a delusional (a false, fixed belief) nature, perceptual distortions, such as auditory hallucinations, lack of volition, affect which is incongruous to the presenting situation, difficulties with attention, speech disorganization, and dysfunction in social and/or occupational situations (APA 1994). It is important to acknowledge that not all individuals with schizophrenia manifest all of the above symptoms, nor do all of these symptoms occur at the same time. The most-used method of classifying schizophrenic symptoms is into positive symptoms in the acute or acute-on-chronic phase, which are hallucinations (sensory ex-perience with no stimulus, e.g. hearing a voice speaking to you when no one is doing so), delusions (a false, fixed belief), a disorganization of speech, or bizarre behaviour, and negative symptoms in the chronic phase, which are alogia (a loss of fluency of thought and speech), blunted affect, apathy, asociality and attention impairment (Andreasen 1989).

Morley and Sellwood (1997) identify two groups of older people with schizophrenia. The first is older people who present for the first time with schizophrenia, which is acknowledged to be rare. The second, which they suggest is a growing population as the number of older people increases, are those who were diagnosed with schizophrenia as young adults and are now 65 years of age or older.

Physical changes as a result of schizophrenia diagnosed in old or very old age are no different to those when it is diagnosed in a younger group, and there is no significant evidence for the development of a dementing disorder (Howard et al 2000). Older individuals are more likely to present with negative symptoms of schizophrenia, such as apathy and withdrawal (Keogh and Roche 1996), which increase the possibility of poor hygiene and nutrition with subsequent physical deterioration. Also, if suspicion of a delusional nature (paranoid delusions) is present, they may place themselves in physical danger, such as locking themselves in their homes and not allowing appropriate help to enter. Because of this, the possibility of suicide must never be ruled out as the last means of escape from disturbing hallucinations or delusions.

Both the positive and negative symptoms of schizophrenia can result in decreased social contact. Positive symptoms of disorganized speech and bizarre behaviour can result in a reduction of their social network, which can sometimes exacerbate their schizophrenic disorder. Symptomatology, such as social disorganization, social dysfunction with relationship difficulties and a lack of emotional reciprocation (APA 1994), can make it difficult to sustain supportive relationships and could potentially result in networks that may be restrictive, disjointed or chaotic (Simmons

1994). In some cases, symptoms of schizophrenia can affect the individual's lifestyle with socially disabling consequences (MacCarthy et al 1989). It is, therefore, likely that supportive contacts will diminish until a core structure remains, usually consisting of professionals, family and illness-related individuals.

Mania/hypomania

A manic episode is thought to begin suddenly and develop over a couple of days (APA 1994). It is distinguished by an abnormally elevated mood, which remains high throughout the course of the illness. There is usually unwarranted irritability and some grandiosity. Speech is pressured with the individual talking very quickly, the sequence of thoughts rapidly changing and only tenuously connected. Individuals are easily distracted and are often in a state of psychomotive agitation. Older people in a manic episode present with similar symptoms to younger individuals, though the period during which they manifest is longer (Cohen et al 1999) and is thought to be milder in form (Keogh and Roche 1996). However, this overactivity – even in this 'milder form' – can put physical strain on systems of the body, e.g. heart, lungs, joints, muscles, etc., which may result in damage and an exacerbation of physical illness. As with the younger age group, physical dangers as a result of overconfident, grandiose or disinhibited behaviour need to be monitored to prevent physical and/or psychological injury.

Often, the overactive, overfamiliar, and overfriendly behaviour of someone in a manic or hypomanic state can result in an increase in social contact, with an 'infectiousness' in their sociability. With older people, this has been found to be both less active and less 'infectious' (Keogh and Roche 1996). However, hostility and resentment are more prominent feelings in this age group, and behaviours, such as displaying a lack of inhibition, can still be distressing to the families involved.

Alcohol dependence

Alcohol dependence can result in deteriorating physical health generally with vitamin deficiency, poor hygiene and poor nutrition. Although once thought to be a small problem with older people, it is now recognized as being more significant. McLoughlin and Farrell (1997) suggest that it is a growing problem with older people as generations from the 1950s onwards reach the age of 65. In a study of older men, Hirata et al (1997) found 15.1% were alcohol dependent and that alcoholism was related to the early development of medical problems and financial difficulties. The question of a genetic component of alcohol dependence is supported by Cook (1996 p. 2), who states: 'There is considerable evidence for a genetic effect on alcohol-related disorders.' However, it is more likely that there is a strong component of learning involved in addictive behaviour, although genetics do have an important role (Vaillant 1995).

It is now recognized that up to 50% of older people with alcohol dependence have some form of mood disorder, such as anxiety or depression (McLoughlin and Farrell 1997). Also, when an older person presents with cognitive impairment, it is necessary to assess whether this is alcohol induced. Again, similar to the younger age group, older people who are actively alcohol dependent behave in a way that is socially restricted and depends upon obtaining alcohol. Their behaviours can be disruptive to families and non-alcohol-dependent friends. Social circles tend to be related to alcohol consumption.

Bio-psycho-social treatments and care

As identified in the introduction to this chapter, there is not enough space to include a discussion of the available treatments and care that may be offered to older people with mental health problems. Table 8.2 lists the main biological and psycho-social treatments and care. Detailed information about these can be obtained by referring to Holmes and Howard (1997), Norman and Redfern (1997) and Woods (1999b).

Table 8.2: Biological and Psychosocial Forms of Treatment and Care

---

Biological Treatment and Care
Medication
Electro-convulsive therapy
Physical health care

Psychosocial Treatment and Care
Psychotherapy
    1. psychodynamic therapy
    2. cognitive behavioural therapy
    3. counselling
Activity-based therapies – music, art, dance, drama exercise, etc.
Reminiscence
Reality Orientation
Validation Therapy
Multi-sensory environments

When considering the most appropriate form of psychosocial care and treatment for clients, it can be helpful to analyse the purpose of a particular intervention and how it might benefit the client. Guidelines for such an analysis can be found in Box 8.3.

Informal care and older people with mental health problems

The previous section of this chapter outlined the main presentations of mental health problems in old age. While a range of treatments and interventions for mental health problems is provided by formal carers, it is interesting to note that informal carers, usually family and/or friends, provide the larger proportion of support to older people with mental health problems (Audit Commission 2000). It has been suggested that home care is given 85% of the time by informal carers (Lyons and Zarit 1999) and that a spouse rather than an adult child is more likely to provide this care (Zarit and Edwards 1999). However, Zarit and Edwards (1999) also note that when an adult child is involved in care-giving, it is usually a daughter. This section will examine informal care-giving and its impact on carers.

Box 8.3: Questions To Consider When Implementing Psycho-social Interventions

What is the overall purpose of this individual/group intervention?
Which client(s) might benefit from such individual/group intervention?
What would be the best size for the group?*
What might be the best structure including overall time span, for the individual/group intervention?
Where will the individual/group intervention sessions be held?
What will be the time of the individual/group intervention and how many per week?
Who will facilitate the individual/group intervention?
What theoretical framework will be used?
Who will support the individual/group intervention used?
What form will the supervision take?

Always ask why with each of these questions, e.g.: 'Why should this client have this type of intervention?'

*For group intervention only.

Although the care-giving role may be taken on by either family or friends, kin relationships are qualitatively different in relation to any feelings of commitment and obligation, with closer relations, such as the spouse or daughters, providing more of the long-term care (Zarit and Edwards 1999). Spouses are usually co-resident with the person being cared for, and it has been identified that the experience of burden and the nature of the relationship with the cared-for person changes when the carer is co-resident (Schneider et al 1999). They found that primary care-giver stress was associated more with behavioural deficits (stubbornness, uncooperativeness and apathy) rather than with behavioural excesses (aggression, restlessness and labile moods). Changes in the spousal relationship between the care-giver and cared-for person can make caring difficult at times, but can also be satisfying. Often communication between partners, an essential part of a successful relationship, is disrupted with reduced reciprocity, even though care-givers continue to involve the cared-for person in decision-making and other daily activities (Sainty 1995). It is interesting to note that in a study by Murray et al (1999), despite a number of difficulties, some spouse carers identified positive aspects of their caring role, such as rewards for their caring, mutual affection and companionship. For example, they found that of the 280 spouse care-givers interviewed, 82% said they received some reward for their efforts.

Informal caring has both a physical and psychological impact on carers. Attending to instrumental caring tasks, such as helping with personal hygiene (especially if there is incontinence), dressing, shopping, housework and general supervision can be physically exhausting. There may also be physical dangers, such as managing aggressive situations. Psychologically, it has consistently been identified that depression is high among informal care-givers of older people with mental health problems (Collins et al 1994). In her study on care-giving demands, Wallhagen (1992) found that care-givers experienced psychological stress because of a constant need to provide care, manage behavioural problems, such as wandering and asocial behaviour, and a lack of communication from the cared for person.

It is also recognized that there is a financial effect on informal caring. The Carers National Association (1994) has drawn attention to the economic costs of providing care. For example, if there is incontinence, the cost of clothing, laundry and incontinence pads needs to be met. In Schneider et al's (1999) study, it was found that 61% of the informal carers had additional expenses because of their caring role, but only 31%

received extra financial assistance, resulting in an expression of dissatis-faction by carers. Although many carers of older people with mental health problems are older themselves and therefore retired, younger family members are also carers and often have to give up work to under-take the caring role. Liken and Collins (1993) provide a vignette of a 47-year-old daughter whose mother had Alzheimer's. In it, she describes having to stop working to care for her mother on a full-time basis, thus incurring financial loss.

Employment not only has an economic role but also a social one. Employment can enhance an individual's social network. However, this changes when becoming an informal carer. In the initial stages of caring, it can also produce role strain because of the multiple roles care-givers undertake and the high level of responsibility in their care-giving role. Zarit and Edwards (1999) highlight the fact that often care-givers leave their employment within three months of taking up their care-giving role. There are other disruptions to social activities, such as at times feeling rejected by family or friends and feelings of social isolation (Schneider et al 1999) as well as a severe limitation in social activities (Koffman and Taylor 1997/1998). Also, family tensions can develop. For example, family conflicts may occur when there are disagreements as to who in the family will be the carer and how this care will be given (Zarit and Edwards 1999).

One way of addressing difficulties experienced by informal carers of older people with mental health problems is through the development of a partnership between formal and informal carers. In order to rectify many of the inconsistencies between what informal carers have said they need and what has been provided, the Carers National Association (1994) has identified a number of principles by which services can be measured. These include a recognition of the skills carers have that can be comple-mentary to the care professionals, to have equal access to services but also choice as to how much they are able to take on the role of informal carer – or even if they want to be carers, they want information, practical help, to be consulted, costs to be kept down and a co-ordination of service, such as at discharge from hospital of the person for whom they are caring. This has been instrumental in government recognition of the important role of informal carers through legislation in the form of the Carers (Recognition and Services) Act 1995 (DOH 1995). However, in *A National Service Frame-work for Mental Health*, it has been identified that the act has not been consistently implemented throughout the country (DOH 1999). However, Soliman and Butterworth (1998) propose a method to encourage full implementation, which is by asking informal carers to participate in the education of formal carers and those who are responsible for implementing policy.

Conclusion

This chapter has identified the prevalence of mental health disorders in the older population. It has been shown that, contrary to stereotypical beliefs about mental illness in old age, depression rather than dementia is the most common problem.

A bio-psycho-social model of the influences and effects of abnormal psychological development in older people has been presented. Although it has not been possible to discuss pharmacological and psycho-social care and treatments, references to detailed sources have been provided. The importance of the role of informal carers in providing care has been identified and explored, recognizing that the impact on informal carers of caring for an older person with mental health problems can be significant.

The overall picture of older people with mental health problems is that they experience the same problems as younger people, though the manifestations may be less active. Also, there are fewer of the severe and enduring mental illnesses, such as schizophrenia, as a first-time problem, in the older age population.

The intention of this chapter has been to offer a balanced account of the mental health problems older people experience and the impact this may have on carers.

References

Abas M (1997) Functional Disorders in Ethnic Minority Elders. In: Holmes C and Howard R (eds) Advances in Old Age Psychiatry pp. 234–245. Petersfield: Wrightson Biomedical Publishing Ltd.

Adams T (1996) Kitwood's approach to dementia and dementia care: a critical but appreciative review. Journal of Advanced Nursing 23 (5): 948–953.

American Psychiatric Association (APA) (1994) Diagnostic and Statistical Manual of Mental Disorders (DSM-IV) 4th edn. Washington DC: American Psychiatric Association.

Andreasen N (1989) The scale for the assessment of negative symptoms (SANS): Conceptual and theoretical foundations. British Journal of Psychiatry 155 (supplement 7): 49–52.

Antuono P and Beyer J (1999) The burden of dementia. A medical and research perspective. Theoretical Medicine & Bioethics 20 (1): 3–13.

Aquilina and Warner (1996) The Royal Free Hospital Handbook of Psychiatric Examination. London: Royal Free Hospital.

Audit Commission (2000) Forget me not: Mental Health Services for Older People. London: Audit Commission.

Ballard C G, O'Brien J, Lowery K, Ayre G A, Harrison R, Perry R, Ince P, Neill D and McKeith I G (1998) A prospective study of dementia with Lewy bodies. Age and Ageing 27 (5): 631–636.

Beekman A T F, Deeg D J H, van Tilburg T, Smit J H, Hooper C and van Tilburg W (1995) Major and minor depression in later life: a study of prevalence and risk factors. Journal of Affective Disorders 36: 65–75.

Blazer D (1993) Depression in Late Life 2nd edn. St. Louis: Mosby.

Brodaty H, Peters K, Boyce P, Hickie I, Parker G, Mitchell P and Wilhelm K (1991) Age and depression. Journal of Affective Disorders 23 (3): 137–149.

Byrne E J (1997) Acute and sub-acute confusional states (delirium) in later life. In: Norman I J and Redfern S J (eds) Mental Health Care for Elderly People pp. 175–182. Edinburgh: Churchill Livingstone.

Carers National Association (1994) A Fair Deal for Carers. Your Guide to Getting Services. London: Carers National Association.

Cervilla J A, Prince M J and Mann A H (1997) The Epidemiology of Alzheimer's Disease. In: Holmes C and Howard R (eds) Advances in Old Age Psychiatry pp. 3–21. Petersfield: Wrightson Biomedical Publishing Ltd.

Cochrane R and Bal SS (1989) Mental hospital admission rates of immigrants to England: a comparison of 1971 and 1981. Social Psychiatry and Psychiatric Epidemiology 24 (1): 2–12.

Cohen R E, Tueth M J and Lenox R H (1999) Psychiatry. Manic behaviour in the elderly. Clinical Geriatrics 7 (7): 38–40.

Collins C, Stommel M, Wang S and Given C W (1994) Care-giving Transitions: Changes in Depression Among Family Care-givers of Relatives with Dementia. Nursing Research 43 (4): 220–225.

Cook C (1996) Genetic factors in drinking disorders. Acoholis: The Newsletter from The Medical Council on Alcoholism 15 (5): 1–2.

Copeland J R M (1999) Depression of older age. British Journal of Psychiatry 174 (4): 304–306.

Copeland J R M, Beekman A T F, Dewey M E, Jordan A, Lawlor B A, Linden M, Lobo A, Magnusson H, Mann A H, Fichter M, Prince M J, Saz P, Turrina C and Wilson K C M (1999) Cross-cultural comparison of depressive symptoms in Europe does not support stereotypes of ageing. British Journal of Psychiatry 174 (4): 322–329.

Copeland J, Dewey M and Griffiths-Jones H (1986) A computerized psychiatric diagnostic system and case nomenclature for elderly subjects: GMS and AGE-CAT. Psychological Medicine 16: 89–99.

Desai M M, Bruce M L and Kasl S V (1999) The effects of major Depression and phobia on stage at diagnosis of breast cancer. International Journal of Psychiatry in Medicine 29 (1): 29–45.

DOH (1995) Carers (Recognition and Services) Act 1995. London: HMSO.

DOH (1999) A National Service Framework for Mental Health. London: HMSO.

Doll R (1993) Review: Alzheimer's Disease and environmental aluminium. Age and Ageing 22 (2): 138–153.

Featherstone M, Hepworth M (1993) Images of Ageing. In: Bond J, Coleman P and Peace S (eds) Ageing in Society: an Introduction to Social Gerontology 2nd edn. London: Sage.

Fitch N (1988) The Inheritance of Alzheimer's disease: a new interpretation. Annals of Neurology 23 (1): 14–19.

Fuentes K and Cox B J (1997) Prevalence of anxiety disorders in elderly adults: a critical analysis. Journal of Behavior Therapy & Experimental Psychiatry 28 (2): 269–279.

Hirata E S, Almeida O P, Funari R R and Klein E L (1997) Alcoholism in a geriatric outpatient clinic of Sao Paulo, Brazil. International Psychogeriatrics 9 (1): 95–103.

Holmes C and Howard R (eds) (1997) Advances in Old Age Psychiatry. Petersfield: Wrightson Biomedical Publishing Ltd.

Howard R, Rabins P V, Seeman M V and Jeste D V (2000) Late-Onset Schizophrenia and Very-Late-Onset Schizophrenia-Like Psychosis: An International Consensus. The American Journal of Psychiatry 157 (2): 172–178.

Katona C L E (1994) Depression in Old Age. Chichester: John Wiley & Sons.

Keogh F and Roche A (1996) Mental Disorders in Older Irish People: Incidence, Prevalence and Treatment. Dublin: National Council for the Elderly, Report Number 45, pp. 63–86.

Kennedy G J, Kelman H R and Thomas C (1990) The Emergence of Depressive Symptoms in Late Life: The Importance of Declining Health and Increasing Disability. Journal of Community Health 15 (2): 93–104.

Kirby M, Bruce I, Radic A, Coakley D and Lawlor B A (1997) Mental disorders among the community-dwelling elderly in Dublin. British Journal of Psychiatry 171 (4): 349–372.

Kitwood T (1990) The dialectics of dementia: with particular reference to Alzheimer's disease. Ageing and Society 10 (2): 177–96.

Kitwood T (1993) Discover the person, not the disease. Journal of Dementia Care 1 (1): 16–17.

Kivelä S-L, Kongäs-Saviaro P, Kimmo P, Kesti E and Laippala P (1996) Health, Health Behaviour, and Functional Ability Predicting Depression in Old Age: A Longitudinal Study. International Journal of Geriatric Psychiatry 11: 871–877.

Koffman J and Taylor S (1997/1998) The needs of carers. Elderly Care 9 (6): 16–19.

Krasucki C, Howard R and Mann A (1998) The Relationship Between Anxiety Disorder and Age. International Journal of Geriatric Psychiatry 13 (2): 79–99.

Lawlor B A, Radic A, Bruce I, Swanwick G R J, O'Kelly F, O'Doherty M, Walsh J B and Coakley D (1994) Prevalence of mental illness in an elderly community dwelling population using AGECAT. Irish Journal of Psychological Medicine 11 (4): 157–159.

Liken MA and Collins CE (1993) Grieving: Facilitating the Process for Dementia Care-givers. Journal of Psychosocial Nursing 31, 1, 21–25.

Lindesay J (1997) Phobic Disorders and Panic in Old Age. In: Holmes C and Howard R (eds) Advances in Old Age Psychiatry pp. 227–233. Petersfield: Wrightson Biomedical Publishing Ltd.

Lobo A, Marcos G, Dia J-L and De-la-Camara C (1995) The Prevalence of Dementia and Depression in the Elderly Community in a Southern European Population. Archives of General Psychiatry 52 (6): 497–506.

Lyons K S and Zarit S H (1999) Formal and Informal Support: The Great Divide. International Journal of Geriatric Psychiatry 14 (3): 183–196.

MacCarthy B, Kuipers L, Hurry J, Harper R and Lesage A (1989) Counselling the relatives of the long-term adult mentally ill. 1: Evaluation of the impact on relatives and patients. British Journal of Psychiatry 154: 768–775.

McKeith I G (1997) Dementia with Lewy Bodies. In: C Holmes and R Howard (eds) Advances in Old Age Psychiatry pp. 52–63. Petersfield: Wrightson Biomedical Publishing Ltd.

McLoughlin D M and Farrell M (1997) Substance misuse in the elderly. In: Norman I J and Redfern S J (eds) Mental Health Care for Elderly People pp. 205–221. Edinburgh: Churchill Livingstone.

Morley M and Sellwood W (1997) Schizophrenia in later life. In: Norman I J and Redfern S J (eds) Mental Health Care for Elderly People pp. 223–245. Edinburgh: Churchill Livingstone.

Murray J, Schneider J, Banerjee S and Mann A (1999) EUROCARE: A Cross-National Study of Co-resident Spouse Carers for People with Alzheimer's Disease: II - A Qualitative Analysis of the Experience of Care-giving. International journal of Geriatric Psychiatry 14 (8): 662–667.

Norman I J and Redfern S J (eds) (1997) Mental Health Care for Elderly People. Edinburgh: Churchill Livingstone.

OPCS (Office of Population Censuses and Surveys) (1993) National population projections: 1991-based. Series PP. 2, Number 18, Appendix 1. London: HMSO.

Orrell M, Butler R, and Bebbington P (2000) Social factors and the outcome of dementia. International Journal of Geriatric Psychiatry 15 (6): 515–520.

Palsson S and Skoog I (1997) The epidemiology of affective disorders in the elderly: a review. International Clinical Psychopharmacology 12 (Supplement 7): S3–13.

Pitt B (1996) Psychogeriatric assessment and management. In: Bryan K and Maxim J (eds) Communication Disability and the Psychiatry of Old Age. London: Whurr publishers.

Pitt B (1997) Defeating Depression in Old Age. In: Holmes C and Howard R (eds) Advances in Old Age Psychiatry pp. 137–142. Petersfield: Wrightson Biomedical Publishing Ltd.

Primeau F (1988) Post-Stroke Depression: A Critical Review of the Literature. Canadian Journal of Psychiatry 33 (8): 757–765.

Prince M J (1995) Vascular risk factors and atherosclerosis as risk factors for cognitive decline and dementia. Journal of Psychosomatic Research 39 (5): 525–530.

Prince M J, Harwood R H, Blizard R A and Mann A H (1997) Impairment, disability and handicap as risk factors for depression in old age. The Gospel Oak Project V. Psychological Medicine 27 (2): 311–321.

Ramsay R, Wright P, Katz A, Bielawska C and Katona C (1991) The detection of psychiatric morbidity and its effects on outcome in acute elderly medical admissions. International Journal of Geriatric Psychiatry 6: 861–866.

Sainty M (1995) In sickness and in health. Journal of Dementia Care 3 (2): 18–19.

Saunders P A, Copeland J R M, Dewey M E, Gilmore C, Larkin B A, Phaterpekar H and Scott A (1993) The Prevalence of Dementia, Depression and Neurosis in Later Life: The Liverpool MRC-ALPHA Study. International Journal of Epidemiology 22 (5). 838–847.

Schaub R T and Linden M (2000) Anxiety and anxiety disorders in the old and very old – results from the Berlin Aging Study (BASE). Comprehensive Psychiatry 41 (2 Supplement 1): 48–54.

Schneider J, Murray J, Banerjee S and Mann A (1999) EUROCARE: A Cross-National Study of Co-resident Spouse Carers for People with Alzheimer's Disease: I – Factors Associated with Carer Burden. International Journal of Geriatric Psychiatry 14 (8): 651–661.

Simmons S (1994) Social networks: their relevance to mental health nursing. Journal of Advanced Nursing 19 (2): 281–289.

Soliman A and Butterworth M (1998) Why carers need to educate professionals. Journal of Dementia Care 6 (3): 26–27.

Stein M B, McQuaid J R, Laffaye C and McCahill M E (1999) Social phobia in the primary care medical setting. Journal of Family Practice 48 (7): 514–519.

Tijhuis M A R, De Jong-Gierveld J, Feskens E J M, Kromhout D (1999) Changes in and factors related to loneliness in older men. The Zutphen Elderly Study. Age and Ageing 28 (5): 491–495.

Vaillant G E (1995) The Natural History of Alcoholism Revisited 2nd edition. Cambridge, Mass: Harvard University Press.

Wallhagen M I (1992) Care-giving Demands: Their Difficulty and Effects on the Well-Being of Elderly Care-givers. Scholarly Inquiry for Nursing Practice 6 (2): 111–127.

Walker Z, Leek C A D'Ath and Katona, C L E (1995) Psychiatric Morbidity in Elderly Attenders at an Accident and Emergency Department. International Journal of Geriatric Psychiatry 10: 951–957.

Woods R T (1999a) Mental Health Problems in Late Life. In: Woods R T (ed) Psychological Problems of Ageing pp. 73–110. Chichester: John Wiley & Sons, Ltd.

Woods R T (ed) (1999b) Psychological Problems of Ageing. Chichester: John Wiley & Sons, Ltd.

Zarit S H and Edwards A B (1999) Family Care-giving: Research and Clinical Intervention. In: Woods R T (ed) Psychological Problems of Ageing pp. 154–193. Chichester: John Wiley & Sons, Ltd.

PART 3
SOCIOLOGICAL

CHAPTER 9

The sociology of later life

KATE DAVIDSON

Introduction

Ageing is a sociologically interesting phenomenon because, although it is virtually a universal experience – almost all of us will get old before we die – it occurs within very diverse and complex social and power dynamic contexts, including socio-economic grouping, health status, access to financial resources, gender, ethnicity and geographical location. For over a century, an ageing population has been on the agenda of social-policy makers in response to the perceived notion of old age as a 'problem' for society, principally the cost to the Exchequer for health, welfare and pension provision. It is paradoxical that, on the one hand, we congratulate ourselves that in our society people live longer than at any other time in history, but, on the other, this section of the population is demonized for costing us so much money. Most research on older people has been grounded in problem assessing and addressing, and as such has pathologized the experience of ageing. It is only comparatively recently that social gerontology has attempted to develop theoretical frameworks that seek to make sense of the experience of ageing.

It is not intended here to provide a comprehensive overview of sociological thought; rather, this chapter outlines the development of sociological theory in the study of ageing and later life and discusses its relevance to current health professional practice. The term 'older people' is used to describe those over the age of 65. The chronology is arbitrary but reflects the statutory age for retirement, which is being equalized to 65 for women and men, phasing in the change from 2010 (Ginn and Arber 1998) (see Note 1 p. 152). In a large, Europe-wide survey, 'old' people were asked what they would like to be called (Walker 1993), and they reported that they preferred 'older people' or 'senior citizens'. What they did not want to be called was 'the elderly'. Earlier texts referenced in this chapter will use 'the elderly' but more recent texts will have stopped using the term. There is frequently a time lag between individual use and general acceptance of language, but, as professionals working with older people, it is important to be aware of these sometimes quite subtle changes.

Why social theory?

If most people were asked, it is likely they would describe sociology as the study of society that tells us what we know already through observation and common sense, but subsumed in an alien vocabulary. In fact, much of what we take for granted in our social world has been moulded by sociological study. 'Action' is not carried out in a social vacuum and the development of social theory has been instrumental in our understanding of why and what we do in professional practice. For example, underachievement of girls in secondary education was investigated by educational sociologists, and this led to 'girl-friendly schooling' policies (Marland 1983). This in turn led to dramatic improvements in exam results for girls and a concomitant rise in tertiary education involvement for women. Similarly, medical sociological input has influenced changing attitudes of professionals to patient involvement in issues such as treatment regimens and pain control (Stacey 1993). Professional healthcare training now emphasizes viewing the patient as a whole person, within a social context, not just as an inflamed appendix or a failed kidney ('the cholecystectomy in Bay 2 needs pain killers'). Sociological investigation of residential care for older people in the 1960s (Townsend 1964) identified the practice of 'warehousing' older people in large residential homes, where they were 'institutionalized' and 'depersonalized'. The terminology becomes more familiar when we know and understand what is being discussed. Interestingly, the word 'carer' emerged in the 1970s in an academic context and filtered through to the general population during the 1980s as a result of the rise of the wider carer debate. Now the word is in common use in a wide variety of contexts.

Traditionally based on the natural science disciplines, it is only comparatively recently that the medical and nursing professions have become more amenable to sociological input to clinical practice (Sharp 1995). The reason for the reluctance to accept social scientific scholarship reflects the historic division in the scholarship of the natural, or 'hard' sciences, and the social or 'soft' sciences.

The discipline of sociology developed in the eighteenth and nineteenth centuries on the coat-tails of the Age of Enlightenment (see Note 2 p. 152), which sought to ask and answer questions about the natural sciences. The pursuit of enquiry into the physical, chemical and biological world that developed 'universal laws' was and, to some extent, still is viewed as the only legitimate scientific scholarship, especially by people who were involved with medical science. This positivist approach considers that sensory observation (empiricism) is the only foundation for the development of scientific knowledge. These methods are applied, for instance, to pharmacological research, where rigorous tests are carried out before a drug can be available for general dispensation. In other words, only by measurement of large but finite numbers of cases, gathered under a wide variety of circumstances, can one infer laws or law-like generalizations that demonstrate reliability, that is the same result will emanate from the same method employed each time. Universal laws are considered to be value-neutral, or value-free, inasmuch as empirical evidence does not take into account any notion of personal agency. For example, empirical research has identified a causal path between poverty and ill health in the UK (Townsend and Davidson 1982, Blaxter 1990, Cooper et al 1999) but does not offer an explanation of individual choices involved with health-risk behaviours. So when investigating the social lives of people, the positivist approach tends towards social-structural explanations, which identify enduring, orderly and patterned causal relationships between elements of society, as distinct from those that refer to human intentions and motives.

From the early 1930s, new schools of thought developed in Chicago and in Frankfurt, which shifted away from the positivistic approach by arguing that value-neutral analysis methods failed to take into account rational reflection upon social, political, cultural and moral values. These sociologists argued that, although value-neutrality is a necessary methodological stance, it is not enough on its own. Sociological investigation should not be seen as just producing an *explanation*, but more than this, an *understanding* of social behaviour. This shift highlighted the value of qualitative as compared with quantitative research methods; that is the interpretation of behaviour through observation and interviewing individuals rather than through analysis of statistical data from which generalizations may be made. There was, and to a lesser extent still is, resistance to these methodologies despite their being over three-quarters of a century old. Discussion on the relative strengths of quantitative and qualitative methodology continues to exercise sociological theorists, but there is a growing recognition of the value of a multi-dimensional approach to research.

Nevertheless, most sociological theory generated before the 1960s was gender, race and age blind, that is societal norms were largely predicated on the lived experience of white males under the age of 65. For example, the generic term 'he' was a given to describe most, if not all, human behaviour. Feminists challenged this male dominated or 'andro-centric' approach and were in turn challenged by people from ethnic minorities who demanded recognition of their cultural diversity. Latterly, social gerontologists have highlighted the way in which age and the life course provide an additional dimension for understanding heterogeneity of social experience.

Gerontology as a discipline

Reflection on ageing is as old as intellectual thought itself. From ancient times, philosophers, scientists, theologians, economists, artists and writers have pondered the meanings and experiences of growing older. However, it was not until the twentieth century that 'gerontology' evolved as a discipline, as discussed below. Gerontology is defined in the *Concise Oxford Dictionary* as 'the scientific study of old age and the process of ageing, and of old people's special problems'. The word derives from the Greek *geron* meaning 'old man'. This is somewhat ironic, given that the majority of people who live to advanced years are female and are more likely to experience problems with health and financial resources. As a result of their biological endowment of a longer life expectancy and the social propensity of men to marry women younger than themselves, women are more likely to be alone when they are old. In the United Kingdom, just under 50% of all women over the age of 65 are widowed as compared to 18% of men. For people over the age of 75, these figures are 65% and 30% respectively (ONS 1998). While women live longer, they also experience more years of limiting long-standing illness (LLSI). In other words they have more chronic sickness and disability than do men and, without adequate pension provision, are more likely to live below the government-specified 'poverty line'. Much of the existing medical and social research on the ageing population has been quantitative, often using secondary data in investigating the health needs and income levels of older people (Victor 1991, Vincent 1995).

Yet, as will be discussed below, there is often a disjunction between governmental statistical reports on the resources, health and living circumstances of older people and how older people themselves view their financial and health status, the ageing process and what being old means to them. In more recent years, however, gerontological theory has reflected mainstream sociological theory, which has moved through a positivistic approach towards compassionate perspectives that better recognize differences in the understanding and interpreting of human behaviour (Jamieson et al 1997).

Old age as a 'problem'

As discussed above, a constant theme in the vast majority of writing on old age, regardless of the discipline or perspective, is one of old age as a problem. The message conveyed by the state and the media is one of an increasing financial burden in health and welfare delivery. Thus, it has been argued, old age is socially constructed as a problem (McMullin 2000). For example, academics who study ageing maintain that the notion of a 'demographic time bomb' and the 'crisis' of a greying population is fundamentally flawed since demographic data offers a projection of population size until the middle of the twenty-first century (Bernard and Phillips 1998). Most would argue that wars, floods and drought could be considered crises, but a situation we have anticipated for over half a century hardly qualifies as an unexpected event (Martin-Matthews 2000). Nevertheless, this crisis ideology is so pervasive that older people themselves equate old age with poverty, infirmity and decrepitude. As a result, many older people, even in their seventies and eighties, do not admit to themselves as being 'old' primarily because they do not perceive their own lives as problematic.

Old age can bring with it special problems of reduced financial resources and age-related diseases, but recent NHS data reveal that the most intensive health and social care is given during the final twelve months of an individual's life (Department of Trade and Industry 2000). A combination of medical advances and environmental improvements in living standards and circumstances has brought about what Fries (1980) terms the 'compression of morbidity'. In other words, more people are living longer and are in better health longer and, therefore, most illness will be concentrated into a short phase at the end of life. Yet all old age continues to be viewed as a time of doom and gloom. What is not often fully understood is the extent to which society influences, and is influenced by, these attitudes to ageing.

Sociological perspectives on the study of ageing

Very early social gerontological theory was developed during the 1930s in the USA and, although rather later and slower, academics in the UK have contributed substantially to the discourse. One of the fundamental problems within the discipline of gerontology is, as has been mentioned already, the enormous diversity in the experience of ageing. Older people are no more or less homogeneous than the rest of the population, their only similarity is in chronological age. There is infinite variety in how people age, according to health and financial status, marital status, gender, ethnicity, housing, geographical location and social support networks. Interest in this multiplicity of factors is indicated by the backgrounds of people who study ageing, from psychology, medicine, and the social, economic and political sciences to practitioners working in private, voluntary and statutory governmental sectors. Furthermore, sociological theory on ageing evolved during the twentieth century and continues to exercise and excite researchers both in academia and the wider community.

Some of the following theories are discussed from the psychological perspective elsewhere in this book, but here I develop the societal rather than the individual perspective of the theory.

Disengagement theory was originally described by Cumming and Henry from a longitudinal study (respondents interviewed over a number of years) of a panel of healthy, financially independent people over the age of 50 in Kansas (US) in the late 1950s. Ageing, according to Cumming and Henry, involves a gradual but inevitable withdrawal from mainstream society in preparation for death.

> Aging is an inevitable mutual withdrawal or disengagement resulting in decreased interaction between the aging person and others in the social system he belongs to. The process may be initiated by the individual or by others in the situation. The aged person may withdraw more markedly from some classes of people while remaining relatively close to others. His withdrawal may be accompanied from the outset by an increased preoccupation with himself; certain institutions in society may make the withdrawal easy for him. When the aging process is complete the equilibrium that existed in middle life between the individual and his society has given way to a new equilibrium characterized by a greater distance and an altered type of relationship (Cumming and Henry 1961 p. 14).

There is a reduction in social interaction, and a loss of the major role in life, usually associated with retirement, and this 'makes room' for younger generations to inhabit the social space. The main criticism of this theory is that it is white male orientated, as exemplified by the wording in the above quote. It does not take into account the experience of women, who are more likely to pass retirement age without 'breaking step', that is whether or not they have exited the labour force, they continue to carry out the majority of the domestic responsibilities. They are also more likely to have worked within the service industries, frequently an extension of traditional domestic female labour, and thus feel less of a disengagement from their pre-retirement existence than men might experience (Arber and Ginn 1993). Women are also more likely to have established a social network of friends, neighbours and family, which they maintain into old age (Jerrome 1996). Men, on the other hand, tend to lose contact with work colleagues when they retire (Thompson 1994). Nor does the disengagement theory recognize the experience of male and female ethnic minorities, who are more likely to work beyond retirement age (Blakemore and Boneham 1995, Vincent 1995). A consequence of the theory is that it legitimizes age segregation and has enabled professionals working with older people to reinforce negative stereotypes and, importantly, devalues the status and self-esteem of those people who do work with and look after older people.

Activity theory offers a perspective completely opposite to disengagement theory. It was primarily developed by Havighurst (1963), who argued that successful ageing involves maintaining, for as long as possible, the activities and attitudes of middle age, including social involvement. Lost roles, such as productivity (contribution to the economy) and reproduction (childbearing/rearing), must be replaced by other activities, such as voluntary work and leisure pursuits. The main criticism is that this is unrealistic and does not take into consideration (or marginalizes) the experience of women, ethnicity or disability, where role replacement, or the maintenance of middle-aged values is frequently not an option. Voluntary work and leisure activities presuppose a certain amount of disposable income and a degree of physical fitness.

There is much merit in the more recent ideological shift away from problem-based perceptions of ageing as a decline and loss, towards a more positive perspective of 'adding life to years', preventing disability and promoting healthy or 'successful ageing'. But we need to be careful. Used uncritically, these ideals can set up a divide between those who are able to diversify and those who cannot, and mirrors the Victorian concept of the 'deserving and undeserving poor'; that is the deserving and undeserving old. Those worthy people who demonstrate self-control and right living will be rewarded with good health and an active life in old age. Those older people who fail to meet the criteria for 'ageing well' are in danger of being stigmatized and blamed for their failing health. In institutional settings, such as a hospital, it is important that health professionals resist judging older people who may have substantial limitations and are already likely to feel disempowered by illness and impairment. How we feel about ourselves is largely determined by how others in society view us.

Symbolic interactionism expounds the theory that it is communication through language and gestures (symbolism) as well as interaction with the physical environment that we understand and locate ourselves in society. We experience our social world through subjectivity (as we see ourselves) and objectivity (as others see us) – as actors and reactors. The ageing process is seen in terms of the relationship between the individual and his/her social environment and the interpretation of events that accompany old age. This is a particularly useful approach in making sense of the ageing process and takes into consideration experience at an individual level. As mentioned above, old age is frequently equated with poor health. It is very important to understand this perspective when nursing older people: these patients view themselves as people who are sick and happen to be old, not that they are sick because they are old. For example, I recall one patient of 86, admitted to hospital with a chest infection, pointing to the other women in the ward and telling me that they were in there because they were old. She, of course, was in hospital because she was sick! The interesting aspect is that probably all the other old women in the ward took a similar view. There is, therefore, a difference between how we view ourselves as individuals and how we view old age generally.

The early 1970s saw the evolution in the USA by Riley et al (1972) of the *age stratification perspective*, which was later developed as the *ageing and society paradigm* (Riley 1988) and is possibly the most cited and utilized approach in the literature on ageing. Its importance lies in the recognition of ageing as a bio-psycho-social dynamic over the life course, that is a combination of biological, psychological and social factors that influence ageing both as process and structure. Fundamental to this perspective is the notion of cohort flow. Most commonly a cohort is defined by year of birth, but it may also be defined in relation to groups of people who experience a significant historical event in different ways. In the UK, the Second World War (1939-1945) is probably the most momentous experience to which older people relate, whether they were children or adults at the outbreak of hostilities. On the other hand, the children of the immediate post-war baby boom (1945-1950) share a birth cohort experience of the development of the welfare state, post-war education, the economic boom periods and the social and moral revolution of the 1960s. Individuals enter and exit roles that are socially learned according to age and age-related expectations and sanctions. These will change over time according to the life-course experience, as indeed will their expectations as patients and clients of health and social services. However, as Riley (1994) points out, there is always a structural lag, because human lives change faster than the social structure.

The *Political Economy of Old Age* is a comparatively recently developed perspective and is defined as the study of the interaction between governmental policy, the economy and old age (Walker 1981, Phillipson 1982). From the politico-economic perspective, the state is thought to reflect the interests of the most powerful members of society and the state acts to maintain its own bureaucratic control. In other words, this is fundamentally a class struggle. The main argument is that old age is essentially structured by policy – retirement age, special benefits for older people, and so on, and is closely allied to the notion of productivity. Central to this is the issue of 'structured dependency' whereby dependency is understood in terms of relationships between the dependent group and the labour market – the exclusion of the majority of older people from the labour market renders most of them dependent on the state for income (Townsend 1981). In the USA, Estes (1979) identifies how the commercial opportunities generated in response to the needs of older adults benefit capital and create an 'aging enterprise', for example the burgeoning of private sheltered accommodation, the business activities of SAGA (holidays, motor and home insurance) and retirement villages/hotel developments in Spain and the Canary Islands offering winter sun. However, Estes (1993) recognizes that this perspective is rooted in the predominantly male experience of employment and economic security and does not adequately address issues of gender and ethnicity, for which a different work pattern means they are often excluded from the labour market long before the official age of retirement.

The most recent development in gerontological thought has been the theory, or rather the theories, of *critical gerontology*, which owes its evolution to mainstream critical theory. It recognizes the importance of the link between theory and practice and is predicated on the understanding of three strands of enquiry. Thus, the knowledge gained through *measurement*, for example health status, care-giving burden, financial resources and so on, complemented by the *compassionate* approach, in terms of understanding the meaning of ageing through literature, personal accounts and reflexivity, together with the *political* approach, which identifies the difference in the effects of gender, class and race, presents a holistic view of the experience of ageing (Achenbaum 1997). The juxtaposition, or interdisciplinariness, of approaches emphasizes the notion of empowerment of older people and, in doing so, grapples with issues of social responsibility and advocacy (Wilson 2000). This removes the spectre of older people as 'burdens' and highlights their contribution to society, not necessarily as wage earners, but as people who fulfil essential functions, such as carers and volunteers, and as such are invaluable citizens in society.

The emergence of critical gerontology reflects the development of feminism. Feminist scholars have challenged conventional wisdom (typically expressed by middle-class white males) and have made deliberate efforts to include the voices and differential experiences of sexuality, race and ethnicity and disability in their discourse (Achenbaum 1997). Like feminism, there is no single brand or strand of critical gerontology that aims to reflect the diversity of experience in old age. The main criticism of critical gerontology is that it seems to be all things to all people and, in being so, does not offer a body of knowledge or theory in the sociologically accepted way. However, Minkler (1996) argues that the combination of measurement, compassion and awareness of 'difference' has the potential for a better understanding of both empowerment and disempowerment in the lives of older people. This in turn has implications for programme development and action research and has particular relevance to health delivery.

As Minkler (1996) points out, health professionals may conduct surveys in a community, for example, using measurable indices such as blood pressure, rates of coronary heart disease and stroke, which can be followed up by health-behaviour-risk counselling. In using this methodological approach, professionals may miss the issues that older people in that community feel are important to their health and well-being, such as inadequate income or the threat of violence in the neighbourhood. They may not have access to 'healthy food' because the local shop (if there is one) does not stock fresh fruit and vegetables, or the older person does not have sufficient resources or is afraid to travel in order to purchase elsewhere. An empowering approach, as exemplified by critical gerontology, would be to work together with older people and help them address the problems that they identify as affecting their health. This critical theoretical approach, although not confined to the study of ageing, has been instrumental in developing the ideological shift from 'top down' to 'bottom up' in power relations between professionals and patients.

Ethnic elders and society

The growing racial and ethnic diversity experienced in the UK is reflected in the small but increasing proportion of ethnic elders. For the majority of non-white elders, the UK is their second homeland. For example, in London, over 90% of non-white people over the age of 65 were born outside the UK and, for over 60%, English is not their first language (Lowdell et al 2000). There are two main groups of non-white elders: black Caribbean who migrated to the UK mainly in the 1950s in response to a call for labour for the post-war reconstruction of Britain, and Indian who migrated mostly in the 1960s for both economic and socio-political reasons. More recent migrants, from Pakistan, Bangladesh and Africa, including those people of Asian origin expelled from Uganda in the 1970s, are generally still below the statutory age of retirement.

Much of the research conducted on ageing, race and ethnicity has been problem-based, concentrating on social inequality and health differentials (Blakemore and Boneham 1995). Early research on race from the USA examined the 'double jeopardy' of growing old and being black in a youth-orientated, primarily white society (Dowd and Bengtson 1978). Norman (1985) writes of the 'triple jeopardy' of being female, black and old. The emphasis on social disadvantage has contributed to the perception of life as an ethnic elder as unrelentingly depressing. Ethnic minority scholars point out that these studies frequently ignore the many strengths in their communities (Minkler 1996). As with the general population, an ageing ethnic population is heterogeneous, and what is required is a research methodology that is sensitive to the diverse cultural experience of ageing within the context of personal history, family and community. Health and welfare delivery is primarily directed at the indigenous UK population and is not always responsive to cultural diversity, such as diet, hygiene protocols, language and power relations. An explicit challenge is to translate rhetoric to reality in empowering a group of people ageing in a second homeland and in an alien culture.

Conclusion

The primary aim of this chapter has been to introduce some sociological theory as it applies to an ageing population. There are many aspects of professional life that are taken for granted, for example, changing power dynamics and cultural shifts, which have been driven by theory generated from sociological and psychological enquiry. While acknowledging that growing older brings special problems for people, I hope to have offered a less pathological account of ageing than you may have hitherto received or perceived. Health status is affected by so many other variables than those that are measured by clinical instruments, and there is infinite variety in how we age. Given that the vast majority of older people with whom you are in contact are in need of medical intervention, it is sometimes difficult to remember that most of us who reach old age are healthy for most of our lives: illness is often compressed into the final few months before death. The ideological shift towards viewing patients in an holistic light and as part of the wider societal experience is encouraging. An important aspect lies in enabling older people to play a greater role in determining a response to their health and welfare needs. However, we still have a way to go in changing the prevailing culture, and it is essential that you, as a professional, are part of this revolution.

Notes

[1.] The Pensions Act 1995: one of the main changes will be the equalization of the state pension age for men and women at 65, phasing this in between 2010 and 2020. Women born before 6th April 1950 will be unaffected (i.e. will continue to be eligible for state pension at age 60) and women born after 5th April 1955 will be 100% affected (i.e. will not be eligible for state pension until age 65).

[2.] The Enlightenment, or Age of Reason, was an eighteenth-century philosophical movement that sought to replace orthodox authoritarian beliefs with rational scientific inquiry. During the seventeenth century, as scientific knowledge increased, such scholars as Newton, Locke, Pascal and Descartes questioned accepted beliefs, and criticism of established society and assumptions spread throughout Europe. In France, philosophers, such as Voltaire, attacked established religion, and the Enlightenment beliefs of individual liberty and equality were embodied in the works of Rousseau and Diderot. New ideas and new approaches to old institutions set the stage for great societal changes, such as those brought about by the French Revolution, and were highly influential in the development of the American Constitution.

References

Achenbaum W A (1997) Critical Gerontology. In: Jamieson A, Harper S and Victor C (eds) Critical Approaches to Ageing and Later Life pp. 16–26. Buckingham: Open University Press.

Arber S and Ginn J (1993) Gender and Later Life: A Sociological Analysis of Resources and Constraints. London: Sage.

Bernard M and Phillips J (eds) (1998) The Social Policy of Old Age: Moving into the 21st Century 1–19. London: Centre for Policy on Ageing.

Blakemore K and Boneham M (1995) Age, Race and Ethnicity. Buckingham: Open University Press.

Blaxter M (1990) Health and Lifestyles. London: Tavistock/Routledge.

Cooper H, Arber S, Fee L and Ginn J (1999) The Influence of Social Support and Social Capital on Health. London: Health Education Authority.

Cumming E and Henry W (1961) Growing Old: The Process of Disengagement. New York: Basic Books.

Department of Trade and Industry (2000) Ageing Population Panel, Report 3: Healthcare and the Older Person Taskforce. London: HMSO.

Dowd J and Bengtson V (1978) Ageing in Minority Populations: An Examination of the Double Jeopardy Hypothesis. Journal of Gerontology 33 (6): 338–355.

Estes C (1979) The Aging Enterprise. San Francisco: Jossey Bass.

Estes C (1993) The Aging Enterprise Revisited. The Gerontologist 33 (3): 292–298.

Fries J (1980) Aging, Natural Death and the Compression of Morbidity. New England Journal of Medicine 303 (3): 130–135.

Ginn J and Arber S (1998) Gender and Older Age. In: Bernard M and Phillips J (eds) The Social Policy of Old Age pp. 142–162. London: Centre for Policy on Ageing.

Havighurst R (1963) Successful Aging. In: Williams R, Tibbitts C and Donahoe W (eds) Process of Aging pp. 311–315. Chicago: University of Chicago Press.

Jamieson A, Harper S and Victor C (eds) (1997) Critical Approaches to Ageing and Later Life. Buckingham: Open University Press.

Jerrome D (1996) Continuity and Change in the Study of Family Relationships. Ageing and Society 16 (1): 91–104.

Lowdell C, Evandrou M, Bardsley M et al (2000) Health of Ethnic Minority Elders in London. London: Directorate of Public Health: 222.

Marland M (1983) School as a Sexist Amplifier. In: Marland M (ed) Sex Differentiation and Schooling. London: Heinemann.

Martin-Matthews A (2000) Intergenerational Caregiving: How Apocalyptic and Dominant Demographies Frame the Questions and Shape the Answers. In: Gee E M and Gutman G M (eds) Apocalyptic Demography and the Intergenerational Challenge pp. 64–79. Toronto: Oxford University Press.

McMullin J (2000) Diversity and the State of Sociological Aging Theory. The Gerontologist 40 (5): 517–530.

Minkler M (1996) Critical Perspectives on Ageing: New Challenges for Gerontology. Ageing and Society 16 (4): 467–487.

Norman A (1985) Triple Jeopardy: Growing Old in a Second Homeland. London: Centre for Policy on Ageing.

ONS (1998) Annual Abstract of Statistics. London: HMSO.

Phillipson C (1982) Capitalism and the Construction of Old Age. London: Macmillan.

Riley M (1988) On the Significance of Age in Sociology. In: Riley M, Huber B and Hess B (eds) Social Structures and Human Lives pp. 24–45. Newbury Park, Calif: Sage.

Riley M (1994) Aging and Society: Past, Present and Future. The Gerontologist 34 (4): 436–446.

Riley M, Johnson M and Foner A (1972) Aging and Society: Vol 3. A Sociology of Age Stratification. New York: Russell Sage.

Sharp K (1995) Sociology in Nurse Education: Help or Hindrance? Nursing Times 91 (20): 34–35.

Stacey M (1993) The Sociology of Health and Healing. London: Routledge.

Thompson E (ed) (1994) Older Men's Lives. Thousand Oaks, California: Sage.

Townsend P (1964) The Last Refuge. London: Routledge and Kegan Paul.

Townsend P (1981) The Structured Dependency of the Elderly: A Creation of Social Policy in the Twentieth Century. Ageing and Society 1 (1): 5–28.

Townsend P and Davidson N (1982) Inequalities in Health: The Black Report. Harmondsworth: Penguin.

Victor C (1991) Health and Health Care in Later Life. Buckingham: Open University Press.

Vincent J A (1995) Inequality and Old Age. London: UCL Press.

Walker A (1981) Towards a Political Economy of Old Age. Ageing and Society 1 (1): 74–94.

Walker A (1993) Age and Attitudes. Brussels: Commission of European Communities.

Wilson G (2000) Understanding Old Age: Critical and Global Perspectives. London: Sage.

CHAPTER 10

Ethical issues associated with ageing

DYMPNA CROWLEY

Introduction

There are ethical issues associated with all stages of ageing, from birth to old age. This chapter will focus on respecting autonomy, giving information to obtain consent and patient decision-making, because these issues are concerned with how older people should be cared for.

Ethics can be described as 'concerning itself with what is right and wrong, good and bad in human actions' (Hendrick 2000 p. 17). An ethical issue is usually recognized because it makes us question the actions of ourselves and others. For the older person, this is most likely to occur when they are in the care of carers and or health professionals. *The Code of Professional Conduct for Nurses, Midwives and Health Visitors* (UKCC 1992) is a set of clauses that reflect the ethical values of professional conduct. These clauses are underpinned by such ethical principles as respect for patients, honesty, promoting well-being, avoiding harm, fairness and maintaining confidentiality.

In caring for older people, we need to examine these values to help clarify the distinction between what our actions are and what they should be. In addition to how we act, we also need to consider how we think. Having the right intention is necessary for ethical conduct as well as acting in the right way (Beauchamp and Childress 1994). However, this is not supported by all of the theories of ethics. Utilitarianism is committed to doing the right action but the motive is unimportant. Deontology, on the other hand, considers the intention of the action to be crucial in determining the morality of the act (Hendrick 2000). It is possible to do the right action but not to have the right intention. The nurse–patient relationship is primarily interpersonal. It follows that the nurse should have the right intention as well as the right action.

Autonomy

This ethical principle recognizes the individuality of people and the need for others to promote individuality. This has a particular significance for older people who may not be able to express their own individuality. The term 'autonomy' comes from the Greek words *autos*, meaning 'self', and *nomos*, meaning 'law'. This self-rule is often expressed as being self-governing, having personal freedom and having individual rights and choices – in other words, being yourself (Beauchamp and Childress 1994). This gives some indication of the importance of the principle with respect to older people, whose ability to be self-governing or to be autonomous may be compromised by physical or mental impairment.

For many writers in healthcare ethics, the principle of respect for autonomy is of primary importance; it governs all other principles and must be respected. If the principle cannot be respected, there is a need to morally justify why this is so. The concept is fairly well defined in ethics literature, but applying it to nursing practice can be complex (McParland et al 2000a).

An autonomous person is able to deliberate, make choices, form and carry out plans (Brown et al 1992, Beauchamp and Childress 1994, McParland et al 2000a). This may seem to be straightforward, but, when applied to some people, it can present difficulties. To always be able to make decisions, formulate plans and carry them out can be difficult for anyone, but, if that person is frail, infirm, or mentally or physically incapacitated, it may not be possible to make choices and execute plans. Dworkin (1988) suggests that autonomy is usually presented as a moral, social or political ideal and in reality is seldom found in the pure form. This suggests that autonomy is open to interpretation and dependent on individual circumstances. The descriptions given are examples of what autonomy is but, as with any individual and any situation, there are individual differences. How people express their autonomy is as individual as how they express their individuality, but autonomy as a moral ideal is a desirable attribute and respect for it should be promoted.

Respect for the autonomy of the individual

To show respect for the autonomy of the individual involves not only respectful action but also a respectful attitude towards the individual. As previously mentioned, according to some ethical theories, it is not sufficient to do a good action; there must also be a good intention (Beauchamp and Childress 1994). This is described as doing the right actions and having proper reasons for doing the actions. When caring for an older person, a situation may develop where an older person is being assisted with some activity of living and, while technically doing the right action, the nurse/carer shows a disrespectful attitude. For example:

> An older woman is getting dressed. A nurse offers assistance but is indifferent to the woman. The woman is not offered a choice of clothing and feels that the nurse would rather not be assisting her.

In addition to respecting the autonomy of the patient, there is an obligation to promote the autonomy of the individual. This includes allowing the patient to choose or not choose, even when these choices seem to go against health and welfare advice. This can often be very difficult for the nurse to accept, for example when a patient refuses treatment that would enhance their quality of life. Patients choosing to go against healthcare advice may need more time spent with them to help them understand the significance of their decision.

Respecting the patient's autonomy is allowing the patient to exercise his or her choice, but the nurse, while accepting this decision, must also accept that the patient may change his or her mind. A patient's present choice may be in conflict with a previous choice. For example:

> An older man accepted drug treatment for high blood pressure but after a few weeks decided that he did not like taking the drugs and did not want to take them for the rest of his life; so he stopped taking the drugs.

The man in this example needs time spent with him to establish his reasons for stopping the medication. Principles of patient education will guide the nurse in exploring these.

It may seem that the choices that are made by patients are not the choices of a person acting autonomously. Beauchamp and Childress (1994) suggest three criteria that can be used to demonstrate autonomous action on the part of the individual. A person acts:

- intentionally
- with understanding
- without controlling influences.

The implications for the older person are that it may take time to establish understanding. Short-term memory declines with age, and the ability to grasp facts and think quickly is perhaps not as sharp as it used to be for the individual. But, as Gray (1994 p. 713) states, 'certain aspects of intelligence decline with age. However, those aspects of intelligence which decline with age, principally short-term memory and the ability to think quickly, are not those aspects of intelligence which allow one to make competent decisions.'

Older people are able to understand information and make decisions. Though it may take longer for them, they should not be precluded from doing so.

In care settings, especially long-term care settings, time is valuable. This may impose unrealistic expectations on staff and present them with obligations that they find hard to meet. Collopy (1988) acknowledges that many competing claims for their time makes it difficult for staff to know how to use the time they have got. A practical solution might be to give the older person some information in writing and some orally, applying the principles of patient education. This helps to achieve respect for the autonomy of the individual.

Authenticity

Some writers suggest that to be autonomous an individual must be 'authentic'. This means actions and decisions should be in keeping with character (Collopy 1988). This may seem a plausible requirement, because if someone says or does something out of character it would seem odd. However, it does beg the question of how well we know anybody to know his or her character. In the context of care for older people, it has major implications. Older people by virtue of their age are likely to be older than their carers and have a lifetime of personal histories and experiences; some will have survived at least one world war and have developed ways of living. This adds up to a personal repertoire that forms part of the individual's character. Chadwick and Tadd (1992) ask whether a carer or even a relative can know a person well enough to be confident that choices and decisions are authentic.

On the other hand, there are situations when it is clear that a person is acting out of character or may not mean what they say. The difficulty with this is that it may sometimes be open to misinterpretation by an anxious or embarrassed carer or relative. There is an ageist argument for not placing too much emphasis on authenticity. If it is used only in care settings for older people and not in all adult healthcare settings, the inequality could be judged as unethical, disregarding the autonomy of the older person. Older people must be seen and accepted for what they are. People change as a result of experiences. Attitudes, behaviours and choices that were once held may be different from the current ones. A person who when young may have argued for the right of everyone to have life saved by the use of life-support technology may now be against the use of such invasive techniques to support his or her own life.

Consent and the older person

Consent to have treatment or not is the means by which a patient exercises autonomy. It can be a perplexing concept; the following broad definition offers a practical application in practice. Consent is the: 'Voluntary and continuing permission of the patient to receive a particular treatment, based on adequate knowledge of the purpose, nature, likely effects and risks of that treatment including the likelihood of its success and any alternatives to it. Permission given under any unfair or undue pressure is not consent' (DOH Welsh Office 1993).

This definition clearly states that knowledge is required about the proposed treatment before consent can be obtained.

Information and consent

The legal case for information to be given before consent can be obtained was established by case law. *Sidaway* vs. *Bethlem Royal Hospital Governors 1985* established the importance of information-giving prior to obtaining consent. This case is centred on a woman who consented to surgery for her neck and shoulder pain. The surgeon told her of the possibility of some risks but failed to tell her of the very small risk of damage to the spinal cord. During the operation, she suffered damage to her spinal cord resulting in severe disability. She sued on the grounds of not been given information about all the possible risks associated with the operation, which meant that she was not able to give informed consent to the operation (Dimond 1995). The case was unsuccessful at the initial trial and before the Court of Appeal. The case went to the House of Lords. The appeal failed because three of the judges applied the 'Bolam Test' to the case to establish if omission of information was negligence.

The Bolam Test was established in *Bolam* vs. *Friern Barnet HMC 1957 2 All ER 118*. This case created the precedent for what would be acceptable and proper professional practice by a body of professional practitioners. It was established that Sidaway's surgeon was not negligent by omitting information about possible damage to the spinal cord.

One other judge, while agreeing that the case should fail, held that the patient had the right to be given information to facilitate informed consent. He applied the 'prudent patient' test. This test was established by an American case, *Canterbury* vs. *Spence 1972 464 F 2d 772*. Giving information is based on what the 'prudent patient' would want to know (Dimond 1995 p. 102). In practice this means establishing with the patient how much information is required before consent is given.

Giving to a patient information that is considered to be acceptable in professional practice could be judged to be utilitarian in its approach. The nurse, by giving the amount of information that is considered to be professionally acceptable, would be acting ethically. Working in partnership with the patient and establishing what the patient wants to know could be judged to be deontological. The nurse's intention is to find out what the patient wants to know and then give the information. In this way, the intention and action are good and therefore ethical.

Competence and capacity

The law recognizes that 'any adult, mentally competent person has the right in law to consent to any touching of his person' (Dimond 1995 p. 88). So, before doing anything for a person, their permission must be sought. The law also recognizes that 'an adult, mentally competent person has the right to refuse treatment' (Dimond 1995 p. 98). In addition to being mentally competent, the adult has to understand the information given. Consent must be given freely and without coercion.

Consent can be given in several forms. It can be implied, such as when a person rolls up their sleeve to have their blood pressure taken. Expressed consent is either in writing, for example the signing of a consent form, or orally, for example when a patient orally agrees to take their medication.

Informed consent and the older person

Informed consent and the older person raises many issues that are both legally and ethically challenging. As can be seen from the definitions above, giving information to enable a person to understand the pros and cons of the proposed treatment is necessary legally. Ethically, it is also necessary, as it demonstrates respect for the autonomy of the individual. The older person may have difficulties with understanding. There may be many reasons for these – poor short-term memory and unfamiliar language are likely to be common contributing factors. Having a poor short-term memory may seem to go against the legal requirements of obtaining a valid consent but, as previously stated, older people can understand information and make decisions.

There are some myths to be dispelled about the psychological aspect of normal ageing. There are minor effects on memory and a slight decline in mental agility needed to solve problems (Watson and Heath 2000). Watson (2000) suggests that the effects on memory, intelligence and personality are minimal and, unless there is an underlying pathology that makes them more severe, they have little effect on the daily life of older people. Health professionals are required ethically, legally and professionally to communicate with people in a language they understand and to establish that they have understood what has been said.

A useful guide is to presume that adults have the mental capacity to make informed decisions until it is proven to the contrary (Masterson 1999). Assessing an individual's capacity to give valid consent can be difficult for a health professional; the following guidelines from the BMA and RCN (1995) are helpful.

In order to have capacity, the patient must be able to:

a. understand, in broad terms and simple language, what the medical treatment is, its purpose and nature, and why the treatment is being proposed for them
b. understand its principal benefits, risks and alternatives
c. understand, in broad terms, the consequences of not receiving the proposed treatment
d. possess the capacity to make a free choice (i.e. free from pressure)
e. retain the information long enough for an effective decision.

Problems in giving information and gaining consent with older people

Health professionals, and nurses in particular, usually provide the patient with information in order to gain consent. This supports patient autonomy and involvement in decision-making. The older person may feel that the professional knows what is best for them and may be reluctant or unwilling to co-operate. Patients, especially older patients in care settings, are known to say that 'you know what is best for me' or ' you can decide'.

Their past experience of healthcare may have given them this impression. Though this may have been the case, times have changed; instead of patients being told what to do, they are increasingly being involved in more decisions about themselves.

However, the professional–personal relationship may impede autonomy and decision-making. Patients can feel the social gap between themselves and doctors, thus inhibiting them from making an informed decision (Buchanan 1995). The patient can be in awe of the doctor and feel that by asking questions they are taking up too much of the doctor's time. Bandman and Bandman (1995) suggest that economic status, social class, education and value differences make equality difficult to achieve. While it is difficult in practice, if the autonomy of the individual patient is to be respected, consideration must be given to the quality of the relationship a healthcare professional has with the patient. The intention of the professional should be directed at the uniqueness of the patient and recognize that they have unconditional worth. Having a nurse involved in doctor–patient consultation can be helpful, as the nurse may be able to answer the patient's questions and clarify what the doctor has said (McParland et al 2000b).

Obtaining consent

The person who is to do the procedure should obtain consent. Therefore, for a medical procedure it would be a medical practitioner, and for a nursing procedure it would be a registered nurse. Most nursing procedures would not require written consent. The consent for such procedures would be oral or implied, for example:

> When a person accepts his/her oral medication or a sleeve is rolled up to allow a blood pressure reading to be taken.

How much information to give

When caring for older people, it is often difficult to know how much information to give a patient, how much they will understand, and whether they will retain the information. Impairment and dependence (BMA and RCN 1995) do not necessarily accompany ageing. Older people are capable of understanding and retaining information. Working in partnership with the patient, applying the legal principle of what the 'prudent patient' would want to know, will help establish what the patient wants to know, how much information should be given and whether the information needs to given in stages. This would also be ethical, as previously suggested. The patient, irrespective of their age, is an individual with individual needs, experiences and expectations. How any nurse relates to any patient is dependent upon the nurse's understanding and use of appropriate communication skills. There will always be situations where the use of these skills will be more challenging in their application than others, for example:

> the patient who refuses to accept that they have a health problem for which they need to take medication for the rest of their life;

or

> the patient who seems to be listening to what is being said but their comments and questions indicate that they have either not been listening or have chosen to ignore what has been said;

or

> the patient who listens to and understands what is being said but who chooses to let the health professional decide.

Such examples are often manifestations of underlying anxieties and not an abdication of responsibility. Supporting such patients and investing in time with them can help them to overcome their anxieties. There are no easy solutions to such problems, but these difficulties should not hinder the nurse from informing the patient and obtaining consent.

Decision-making and the older person

Decision-making is linked to an individual acting as an autonomous person. Decision-making should be part of any interaction the nurse has with the patient. However, the experience of caring for older people highlights difficulties that can be encountered when decisions have to be made.

In the past, patients were expect to be passive recipients of healthcare, including nursing care. They were regarded as being unable to make decisions about their care (Biley 1992) and therefore not involved. Nursing encouraged and promoted dependence in the patient. Nurses were trained to 'do' for patients. In recent years, there has been a change in the thinking concerning the role of the nurse and consequently that of the patient. This is tied in with many influences that have questioned nursing practice and attitudes to patients. The promotion of individualized care, working in partnership, the increasing movement towards consumerism, and greater knowledge of health issues, has done much to shift thinking and practice. These changes have also been influenced by ethical, legal and social factors. Ethically, healthcare is moving from a culture of paternalism to that of promoting patient autonomy. Legally, the shift is from consent to informed consent, and, socially, from a passive recipient of healthcare to a consumer of healthcare. Laudable as these influences are on healthcare practice, the experience of nursing practice and evidence from the litera-ture suggest that these changes are accompanied by problems.

Older people who require healthcare are more than likely to have had previous experiences of healthcare. These people are now expected to make decisions which in the past were made by health professionals. Patients can be distressed by having to decide. In addition to the previ-ously identified statements that patients make, expressions like 'I don't know what to do' should make the nurse stop and think about what may be behind this and other expressions. The patient may feel unable to make a choice or decision, or may feel that they need the nurse's assist-ance to do so.

Involvement in decision-making is to be encouraged for the reasons already given, but involvement could have the opposite effect to that which is intended. Waterworth and Luker (1990) found that patients like to 'toe the line' because they are so concerned about fitting in. They may feel that they have no rights when dealing with a healthcare professional. Fitting in, pleasing the nurses and not wishing to be a nuisance, they will do as they are told. It seems that encouraging what is considered to be good practice, that is promoting patient participation, may unwittingly coerce patients into doing something that they are unwilling, or unable, to do. Involving patients in decision-making is not about promoting good practice over the individual needs of the patient. Ethically, the focus is on the patient, and an emphasis on the individual needs of patients takes precedence over the promotion of a specific area of practice. Promoting autonomy and independence could be viewed as objectives of nursing care, without compromising the individuality of the patient.

Some patients may not wish to make decisions. There may be several underlying factors that contribute to this. Davies et al (1997) suggest that the research in patient participation has failed to consider factors such as the patient's educational background, age, gender and diagnosis. These may have an effect on whether patients wish to be involved in decision-making or not. The limitations of knowledge should not belie the ethical obligations nurses have when working with older people. Decision-making can be a difficult and vexing prospect for anyone. Allowing time, if it is possible to do so, can remove some of the pressure a patient may feel initially. This time could give the patient an opportunity to ask questions, clarify uncertainties and perhaps help them to feel in control. Enabling patients to make choices and participate in decision-making are fundamental in nurse–patient interactions. Biley's (1992) study found that giving patients control of even a small aspect of care can be beneficial to them. These small beginnings may eventually enable the older person to gain control and increase their participation in decision-making.

This is not a panacea for promoting all decision-making. There will be constant ethical, legal and professional challenges encountered when caring for older people. For example, patients with cognitive impairment, loss of hearing, and impaired vision or speech may be denied adequate involvement and support in making decisions about their care and treatments. Health professionals should not assume that decision-making cannot be achieved, but should accept that patients may fluctuate in their ability to make decisions (Masterson 1999). The emphasis of care should be on maximizing the patient's ability to make decisions. This can be achieved in several ways. The (BMA and RCN 1995 p. 11) checklist is a helpful guide:

- Assess the capacity to make decisions on a decision-making basis and do not make assumptions about competence before adequate assessment.
- Appreciate that incompetence in one area of decision-making does not necessarily mean incompetence in another.
- Delay decision-making until an opportunity presents itself, for example a lucid phase.
- Allow time for the person to make decisions.
- Written information about the risks and benefits of treatment can help overcome poor memory, allow people to review and reinforce what they have been told and to reflect on the issues in their own time.
- Work to understand the individual's values and how the person would wish to live; this understanding can arise from understanding an individual's biography and values, and may also arise from day-to-day relationships.

- Do not assume that the older person's values are the same as your values.
- Emphasize functioning rather than diagnosis.
- Permit the person to choose and facilitate that choice.
- Avoid transferring decision-making to relatives when the patient has not been included in the process.

The end result will be that the patient will either make a decision or not make a decision. In doing the latter, the patient, it could be argued, is exercising autonomy by allowing the decision to be made by another. The nurse has to act in the patient's best interest. The UKCC (1996) advises that acting as an advocate for the patient is respecting their decision. 'Respect for patients' and clients' autonomy means that you should respect the choices they make concerning their own lives' (UKCC 1996).

Conclusion

This chapter has focused on some key ethical issues that make a difference to the care and well-being of older people. Respecting autonomy, giving information, obtaining consent and involving patients in decision-making are shown to be important and special in dealing with older people. When it is not clear what to do when faced with a difficult ethical situation, it seems that the best approach to pursue is to work with the patient and, when this is not possible, work on collaborating with the patient's family to promote the patient's best interests.

References

Bandman E L and Bandman B (1995) Nursing Ethics through the lifespan 3rd edn. London: Prentice Hall International.

Beauchamp T L and Childress J F (1994) Principles of Biomedical Ethics 4th edn. Oxford: OUP.

Biley F C (1992) Some determinants that affect patient participation in decision-making about nursing care. Journal of Advanced Nursing 17 (4): 414–412.

BMA and RCN (1995) The Older Person: Consent and Care. London: British Medical Association/Royal College of Nursing.

Brown J M, Kitson A L and McKnight T J (1992) Challenges in Caring: Explorations in Nursing and Ethics. London: Chapman & Hall.

Buchanan M (1995) Enabling patients to make informed decisions. Nursing Times 91 (18): 27–29.

Chadwick R and Tadd W (1992) Ethics and Nursing Practice A case Study Approach. London: Macmillian Education Ltd.

Collopy B (1988) Autonomy in long-term care: some crucial distinctions. The Gerontologist 28 (Supplement issue): 10–17.

Davies S, Laker S and Ellis L (1997) Promoting autonomy and independence for older people within practice: a literature review. Journal of Advanced Nursing 26 (2): 408–417.

Department of Health, Welsh Office (1993) Code of practice, Mental Health Act 1983. London: Department of Health.

Dimond B (1995) Legal Aspects of Nursing 2nd edn. London: Prentice Hall.

Dworkin G (1988) The Theory and practice of Autonomy. Cambridge: Cambridge University Press.

Gray M J I (1994) The Health Care of the Elderly. In: Gillon R (ed) Principles of Health Care pp. 711–731. London: Wiley.

Hendrick J (2000) Law and Ethics in Nursing and Health Care. Cheltenham: Stanley Thornes.

Masterson A (1999) Frail and vulnerable older people. In: Heath H and Schofield I (eds) Healthy ageing: nursing older people pp. 319–338. London: Mosby.

McParland J, Scott P A, Arndt M, Dassen T, Gasull M, Lemonidou C, Valimaki M and Leino-Kilpi H (2000a) Autonomy and clinical practice 1: identifying areas of concern. British Journal of Nursing 9 (8): 507–513.

McParland J, Scott P A, Arndt M, Dassen T, Gasull M, Lemonidou C, Valimaki M and Leino-Kilpi H (2000b) Autonomy and clinical practice 3: issues of patient consent. British Journal of Nursing 9 (10): 660–665.

Waterworth S and Luker K A (1990) Reluctant collaborators: do patients want to be involved in decisions concerning care? Journal of Advanced Nursing 15 (8): 971–976.

UKCC (1992) Code of Professional Conduct for the Nurse, Midwife and Health Visitor. London: UKCC.

UKCC (1996) Guidelines for Professional Practice. London: UKCC.

Watson R (2000) Normal ageing. Elderly Care 12(2): 23–24.

CHAPTER 11

Ageing in minority ethnic groups

MARY TILKI

Introduction

At the turn of the twenty-first century, there is increasing awareness in Britain of the inadequacy of health and social services provision for older people from minority ethnic groups (Blakemore 2000, Evandrou 2000, Lowdell et al 2000). There is generally wider recognition of the need to develop accessible and culturally appropriate services. However, the absence of adequate data, the complexity of ethnic identity and a lack of clarity about what constitutes cultural competence make planning and evaluation difficult (Parekh 2000).

The chapter is influenced by a number of transcultural theorists and is underpinned by the model of transcultural-skills development proposed by Papadopoulos et al (1998). This approach takes a different perspective from other models, beginning with a focus on the culture of the practitioner and going on to recognize the complexity of ethnic identity, the heterogeneity within any group and the similarities between different groups. The authors particularly acknowledge the existence and effects of institutional racism and the role of professionals in addressing them. The model suggests four levels of skills acquisition beginning with cultural awareness, moving to cultural knowledge and sensitivity, and culminating in cultural competence. Although this chapter relates to older people, many of the issues are applicable to the minority ethnic population as a whole.

Cultural awareness

The importance of cultural self-awareness is exemplified in the difficulties arising from the broad classification of ethnicity used in the census and other datasets and in much of the professional literature. As an example, the term 'Asian' masks a range of differences about the people it purports to describe. People referred to as 'Asian' come from countries like India, Pakistan and Bangladesh and from a range of religious backgrounds, belong to different linguistic communities and social traditions and have had different experiences in Britain. Some will have spent time in second countries such as Uganda or other parts of East Africa and will have been exposed to different cultures and traditions as a result. Similar diversity exists within other minority ethnic groups and, indeed, within the classification of the majority population of the UK. The classification of ethnicity represented in national census data demonstrates the limitations of British ideas of ethnicity that are based solely on skin colour. Although the 2001 Census categories address this to some extent, the neglect of the ethnicity of people from minorities who are not black, and the various ethnicities within indigenous British society, remains a problem. The definition of 'ethnicity' used in this chapter will be that recommended by the London Race, Health and Social Exclusion Commission (Association of London Government 2000) and will include both visible and invisible minority ethnic communities.

Recognizing how we perceive our own ethnicity and the extent to which we identify with one or more cultures is a crucial starting point for understanding other people. Acknowledging our own socialization, the extent to which we adhere to familial and cultural traditions can encourage us to consider the complexity and contextual nature of our own ethnic identity. Examining the context within which we select or reject elements of our own culture, adopt aspects of others and change with time can enable us to see our own cultural identity as dynamic and multifaceted. This should help us to avoid labelling people under rigid ethnic categorizations, and it should encourage us to see differences as variations of normal, rather than as abnormal or problematic.

Although older people from different minority ethnic groups have much in common with each other and with the majority older population, there is little evidence of homogeneity within this cohort. Labels like 'Asian' or 'Caribbean' not only neglect differences in birthplace, religion and language but also deny the impact of migration on individuals. People from different minority ethnic groups, men and women, single people and those with families, will have had differing experiences of migration and varying positions in the labour market. The impact of wider social factors on material resources and subsequently on health will be varied. People will have retained elements of their own heritage and tradition and adapted with varying degrees of willingness to aspects of

British culture. In old age, there will be a range of feelings about 'home' with some still wishing to return to their place of origin while others having little hesitation about staying.

Cultural knowledge

Although cultural awareness enables us to have an open mind about people from cultures other than our own, cultural knowledge is essential if we are to understand the experience of different communities. Knowledge in itself does not guarantee appropriate care, but a lack of understanding of cultural need, barriers to access, or health beliefs and practices may lead to insensitive and poor-quality care.

Limitations of existing data

There is an absence of accurate statistical data on the numbers of older people from minority ethnic groups in Britain, and this is compounded by the inconsistent and sometimes inappropriate use of categories. It is difficult to provide accurate information or comparisons when, for example, one study uses the term 'Caribbean' and another refers to 'Afro-Caribbean'. The term 'black', while being positive for some groups, belies the heterogeneity of experience and status of people from Africa, the Caribbean, and countries of the Indian sub-continent. Despite many shared experiences, people from India, Pakistan and Bangladesh reject the use of the term 'black', and in more recent literature are referred to as 'South Asian'. Likewise, the inclusion of many different ethnic groups in the 'white' category assumes homogeneity with the indigenous population. The scope of this chapter does not allow for a full discussion of the complexity of ethnic classification, but the reader is referred to the work of Aspinall (1999, 2000), Modood et al (1997) and Parekh (2000). However, while research in the future must look towards investigating the experience of different communities (Aspinall, 1999, 2000), most existing evidence about minority ethnic groups is based on aggregated census categories.

Although the requirement to maintain ethnic monitoring records is now mandatory, there is still a persistent failure by health and welfare authorities to collect these data. While ethnicity is monitored more frequently in local authority and social services departments, the picture is still patchy, and there is little evidence to say that the information is used effectively (SSI 1998, Pharoah 1995). Even where NHS data are kept, the categories recorded are often inadequate and poorly organized (Aspinall 1999). The absence of data in primary care is particularly notable, given the role of this sector in providing services for older people.

The failure to collect specific statistics for white minorities means that there is an absence of evidence with which to demonstrate disadvantage or need. Consequent on this failure is the absence of, or at best limited strategic planning for, the needs of white minority ethnic groups despite large numbers in certain parts of the country. Although to some extent this was addressed in the 2001 Census, time is running out for the older people from white minority communities who have contributed so much to this society.

Existing data provide limited information on morbidity or the experience of ill health or service use. The focus on a few specific diseases has led to a neglect of common problems like heart disease, diabetes or hypertension. There are few data on economic resources in later life (Evandrou 2000). Some groups have been studied fairly extensively, while others have been largely neglected. There is a relative dearth of information about older people from minority ethnic groups or their carers. The failure to take account of issues of class, generation or gender in research studies may lead to assumptions that problems arise from the cultural or ethnic background of the individual or community. The blame is then focused on the person or the group rather than on factors such as low income, poor housing, lack of local resources or the inadequate provision of primary-care services.

Demographic trends

While there are numerous problems with data on minority ethnic groups, it is still clear that there are increasing numbers of older people from minority ethnic groups in the population of the UK. In 1996/7 older people from minority ethnic groups comprised just over 6% of the population, but by 2011 this will have reached somewhere in the region of 17% (Aspinall 2000). However, looking at overall national figures belies the fact that minority ethnic groups are concentrated in specific parts of the UK, particularly in inner-city areas. In 1991 non-white people formed 15.1% of the over-65s population of the London Borough of Brent, but by 2001 this had doubled, with the largest increases in the Caribbean and Indian groups (Lowdell et al 2000). Although the over-65s population of London is lower than elsewhere in England and Wales and is likely to reduce (Lowdell et al 2000), it is estimated that the numbers of older people from minority ethnic groups will increase threefold from 1991 to 2011. As with the rest of the population, women generally outnumber men at older ages. However, in the Pakistani and Bangladeshi communities, the number of men is more than twice that of women and to a lesser extent in the Indian and Caribbean communities (Evandrou 2000).

More recently, there has been timely acknowledgement that the 'White' census category comprises large and distinctive minority ethnic communities, such as the Irish and people from places like Cyprus and Turkey (Evandrou 2000, Association of London Government 2000). Despite a lack of accurate figures, it would appear that there are increasing numbers of older people from white minorities living in distinctly localized communities in the UK (Lowdell et al 2000). Unlike other ethnic minorities, elderly Irish people already exist in large numbers in all the post-pensions age bands as well as a significant proportion in the pre-pension age group who will add substantively to the overall numbers in the future (Tilki 1998a, Evandrou 2000).

Social and socio-economic factors

There are differences within and between minority ethnic groups in the access to material and social resources (Evandrou 2000). Some of the differences in housing tenure and living patterns in earlier life are continued in old age. Elders of Pakistani, Bangladeshi, Caribbean and Irish origin are respectively in the lowest-income quintile of the population (Evandrou 2000). A low proportion of minority elders are in receipt of a pension from their former employer and are more likely to be in receipt of income support.

A significant proportion of Pakistani, Bangladeshi, Caribbean and Irish elders experience multiple deprivation compared to the white or Indian Populations. South Asians (people from India, Pakistan or Bangladesh) are twice as likely to live in multi-generational households than are either the white or Caribbean populations. Older Caribbean people are more likely to live in social housing and Pakistani and Bangladeshi elders tend to live in overcrowded accommodation without central heating. Contrary to commonly held assumptions, the average number of children is low in Irish and Caribbean households, and in both communities older age people are more likely to live alone.

However, Blakemore cautions against the presumption that all minority ethnic groups are disadvantaged or problematic and cites examples of affluence in the East African Asian (those who left East Africa during the reign of Idi Amin) and Indian communities (Blakemore 2000).

Access to health services

Data on access to health services are patchy and conflicting. Analysis of general practitioner (GP) consultation suggests that, even when controlled for factors such as limiting long-term illness (illness that restricts daily living), older people from some groups consult their doctors more frequently than do their white counterparts (Lowdell et al 2000). Patterns of access to hospital and GPs vary, and family-doctor and outpatient services are used in different proportions by men and women and by people from some groups rather more than others (Smaje 1995, Lowdell et al 2000). The National Survey of General Practice shows that people from minority ethnic groups have a poorer-than-average experience with their GPs across a range of indicators (NHSE 1999). The higher use of GP services is not reflected in outpatient referrals, and suggests that the rates of consultation may well reflect the dissatisfaction with outcome (Nazroo 1997).

There is limited evidence relating to the uptake of day care, home care, meals on wheels and other community-based services, but the data that do exist suggest neglect by health and social services. The religious and cultural needs of small minority ethnic groups and white minorities are particularly unlikely to be considered in Community Care Plans (Evandrou 2000, Lowdell et al 2000). Although there is little information about the availability or quality of services for people from minority ethnic groups who are terminally ill or dying, there is some evidence that cultural insensitivity and poor care are responsible for much distress to Caribbean people and their relatives (Addington-Hall 2000). Although some genuine attempts are being made to ensure that services are relevant – accessible and good examples of practice and service delivery do exist – the variety of services and the choice to older-age people from ethnic minorities is limited (SSI 1998).

There is evidence of difficulty in gaining access to services, owing to poor health, transport, cost and a lack of information about availability (Boneham et al 1997, SSI 1998). There is reticence about using services that are not sensitive to cultural, religious, dietary or linguistic needs (Brownfoot 1998, Jewson et al 2000). Many older clients do not particularly desire culturally specific services, or care who provides them, as long as those who do are sensitive to their cultural needs (Brownfoot 1998, Jewson et al 2000, SSI 1998). Although some groups do not necessarily want culturally exclusive provision, it is clear that some feel more comfortable within their own community (Brownfoot 1998, Tilki 1998a).

Familial-care networks

Studies throughout the 1980s and early 1990s have shown that health and social services were inaccessible to people from minority ethnic groups (Pharoah 1995). The Social Services Inspectorate (SSI 1998) found that, although most community-care plans and community-care charters made statements about the *needs* of people from minority ethnic groups, there were less specific statements about any actual *actions* to meet these needs. Effective consultation was patchy and the needs of smaller groups, like the Chinese, were rarely considered. Despite a wealth of information about ethnic elders, this evidence was not used in service planning.

It is commonly assumed that older people from minority ethnic groups have a large and supportive family who are willing and able to care for them (SSI 1998). This belief neglects differences in the migration patterns of minority ethnic groups, which results in a significant proportion of older people living alone with few social contacts (Tilki 1998a, 1998b). This idea fails to acknowledge how the availability of housing, patterns of co-residence, low income and multiple deprivation affect the ability of the family to care (Blakemore 2000).

There is also a tendency to presume that familial care facilitates independence and prevents isolation and marginalization. In Leicester, Jewson et al (2000) have shown that the outward migration of Asian families from the inner city to suburban areas disrupted the social networks of older people and left them isolated for long periods. Cultural convention, language difficulty and adverse climate cause many to feel incarcerated and abandoned in the home as the family go about their daily business (Jewson et al 2000). Blakemore (2000), comparing support for Afro-Caribbean and Asian elders in 1985 and 1999, suggests that the inevitability of social change leads to a need for differing approaches to community support. Recent responses indicated that older people were experiencing greater isolation and perceived that the family was disintegrating. However, emerging from this change were extra-familial ways of meeting need, such as culturally specific sheltered housing developments and residential accommodation. Although the stigma of using community or institutional services can prevent some families from seeking help (Brownfoot 1998), it is clear that patterns are beginning to change (Blakemore 2000).

Although familial care can be warm and supportive, it is not inevitably so in any community. The expectations of the community, the elder and the carer lead to a sense of obligation, which may not be the best foundation for a caring relationship. There is a need to consider the roles played by different family members, and particularly the demands placed on women. The reality of being a carer in an extended family network in Jamaica or the Punjab is a very different experience to that in an English city, where there may be a limited group of relatives and friends to share the task of caring.

Although as yet the evidence is limited, there is little attention to the potential abuse of older people from minority ethnic communities (SSI 1998). Recurrent anecdotal accounts of elder abuse in minority communities are emerging (SSI 1998), and research is needed to identify predisposing factors and preventive strategies.

Health status

Higher proportions of people from Pakistan, Bangladesh and the Caribbean report their health as being fair to poor, even allowing for socio-economic status (Nazroo 1997). The incidence of limiting long-term illness (that which restricts daily living) is higher in minority ethnic groups, even when age is taken account of, with Pakistani, Bangladeshi and Irish people having a greater incidence than other groups. There is a range of common health problems that are known to occur in people from different minority ethnic groups. Coronary heart disease is high in South Asians, Irish and people from African and Caribbean groups. Hypertension and stroke levels are increased particularly in people from Caribbean, South Asian and Irish communities. Diabetes is high in South Asian and Caribbean groups, and, although there is a lack of data, there is anecdotal evidence of a greater prevalence of the disease amongst people from Cyprus. Diabetes has a disproportionate effect on older people from some minority ethnic groups who experience the long-term effects of renal problems, diabetic retinopathy, eye disorders, neurological and circulatory complications. With the exception of the prostate, levels of cancer are generally lower in black and Asian communities, although Irish people have the highest incidence of all cancers in the population as a whole (Harding and Allen 1996).

Much of the research on mental illness has focused on younger age groups, specific communities and categories of illness (Lowdell et al 2000). It is argued that the mental health of all older people is a neglected area (Hancock 1998, Jones 1998). Despite some local research (Boneham et al 1997, McCracken et al 1997, Brownfoot 1998) there is a particular neglect of older people from minority ethnic groups (Ebrahim 1996, Rait et al 1996). Although it is acknowledged that there are problems with assessment tools (Boneham et al 1997, Ebrahim 1997), there is an urgent need to investigate the incidence of depression, dementia and other disorders in older age groups. Given the impact of socio-economic factors and isolation due to language and health limitations, it is possible that ethnic elders have high rates of depression. The incidence of dementia rises with age, and there is evidence that it exists in minority ethnic groups, but there is a reluctance to use the services that are offered (Boneham et al 1997, Brownfoot 1998). There may well be a similar reluctance to seek help for depression or other mental health problems.

Health beliefs

Although there is limited research on health beliefs in older people, and particularly those from minority ethnic groups, the evidence from the general studies is applicable. People from working-class origins tend to describe health in relation to the ability to perform daily activities, while those from the middle-classes emphasize more psychological aspects (Calnan 1987, Stainton-Rogers 1991). A number of authors cite low expectations of health in old age as well as a moral imperative to cope and not to give in (Blaxter and Patterson 1982, Cornwell 1984, Sidell 1995). One study of Asian and Caribbean people in East London demonstrated a degree of fatalism about poor health while still attributing it to behaviour, germs, viruses and worry (Donovan 1986). External matters were seen as common causes of ill health and, with the weather, housing, pollution contributing to, or prolonging, colds and fevers. There was also widespread support for the use of folk remedies in the prevention or relief of illness. Such beliefs could also reflect dissatisfaction with, or the inability to use, conventional health services.

However, because healthcare beliefs reflect the society in which they occur, people from minority ethnic groups are likely to share many of the values of the majority culture. They too will wish to avoid the indignity of disability and perceptions of dependence. However, adjustments to ageing, illness and disability are influenced by the presence of social networks, the adequacy of housing and the availability of income. This suggests that, while some older people such as those from the East African Asian community may be at an advantage in all three areas, others, like the Bangladeshi or Irish communities, are disadvantaged.

Cultural sensitivity

Cultural sensitivity in practice settings relies on the cultural awareness, knowledge and particularly the commitment of individual practitioners.

Culturally defined practices around visiting, prayer and diet pose a challenge to the ritual and routine of a hospital or residential setting. Unless the organization makes provision of relevant facilities for prayer, diet and language, it can be very difficult to deliver culturally sensitive care. Although there is no blueprint for any group, empathy, respect and trust provide a good foundation for high-quality care.

Empathy

Empathy is an important attribute and relies on understanding how minority ethnic older age people may feel about spending the last years of their life in a different homeland. The majority of migrants came to Britain in the 1950s and 1960s to work, to better themselves and to return home after a limited time (Byron 1999). A combination of low incomes, high rents and the formation of families and a material commitment to the family back home meant that immigrants were forced to delay thoughts of returning home until retirement. It has been argued that the dream of return helped them to survive difficulties and disadvantage by diverting dissatisfaction into the hope of return (Blakemore and Boneham 1994). However, although many would like to live in another country not all make plans to return home (Byron 1999, Bhalla and Blakemore 1981). For many, changes within themselves, the family and the home society give a sense that they are no longer a part of the society they left. The availability of an index-linked UK pension, a house to sell, the waiving of customs duties and the opportunity for economic activity are all important matters that affect their ability to return home successfully (Byron 1999). The obligation to support children and grandchildren, the unwillingness to lose health care and other advantages of life in the UK and the dispersal of the family at home prevent a number of people from returning to their homeland. Some will be content with the decision to stay, but for others the wish to return is strong, and the realization that they may never see home again is painful.

Respect

Respect is central to establishing trust. It relies on a commitment to value and a willingness to accept beliefs and practices that may be different to those we hold personally, and which may be incongruous with the routines and rituals of the health care system. Many older people from all walks of life regret what they see as the lack of respect afforded them in present society. However, many ethnic elders see this as a reflection of Western values and may be anxious about being abandoned by their families and community. As in all cultures, the need for privacy and dignity are crucial, but a special effort to show respect is necessary when people already feel undervalued in the host community. Trust may be hard to establish for people who have experienced hostility and discrimination in their lives, but respect offers a sound foundation on which it can be established.

Interpersonal skills

Although respect is a complicated concept, there are expectations of the way in which it is demonstrated in different communities. For the majority, the mode of address and greeting conventions are important. Older Caucasian people will generally prefer to be addressed as 'Mrs' or 'Mr' unless they give permission to use the first name, and the same applies to other ethnic groups. Each community will have its own convention, with some using the relevant translation of 'Mrs' or 'Mr' or another title with the first name or family name. Others will use the translation of 'Aunt' or 'Uncle' with or without the name. Greeting customs vary, but it is important to recognize that the eye contact so valued in British society is disrespectful in many cultures, especially when talking to older people or those in authority. Much can be learned from the client, the family and particularly from colleagues from other cultures (Tilki et al 1994).

Communication

While language can be a real barrier to effective care, the commitment of the practitioner and the willingness to communicate are more important and are central to respect for the human being. Although language can be a problem for clients, families and professionals, it is all too easy to rely on formal or informal interpreters and to avoid attempting to improve communication. Many older people who have been in Britain for years understand English but lack the confidence or the speed to use it when unwell. Given time, a trusting relationship and a degree of creativity, older people can be encouraged to use the words they have more effectively.

Reversion to a first language after years of using a second can be a symptom of both physical and mental illness. After any acute illness, or following a stroke, people may lose some or all of their ability to speak English. Dementia can lead to a loss of the ability to speak or understand despite years of fluency in the second language. Those who are not fluent or confident about their English may understand it and, given adequate time and sensitivity, may be able to communicate relatively effectively. Staff who take the trouble to learn words and phrases phonetically will be able to communicate more effectively and may also enjoy their new skills.

Cultural competence

There is evidence that nurses lack sensitivity and skill in delivering culturally appropriate care (Askham et al 1995, Gerrish 1999, Patel 1999). Cultural competence may be easier for staff who share either the cultural background of the client or the experience of migration. However, it may be developed through the use of biographical and reminiscence approaches to care and therapy (Tilki 2000). A biographical approach to the care of older people relies on understanding the client's life history (Johnson 1976) and is particularly pertinent to people from minority ethnic groups whose life story may be unfamiliar to the practitioner. Using the principles of reminiscence to underpin practice can be particularly effective for all clients, and especially those from minority ethnic groups (Tilki 2000). These approaches can enable practitioners to understand a neglected group of people who are coming to terms with growing old in a society where age is devalued, there is increasing xenophobia, and widespread institutionalized racism.

Assessment

A combination of biographical and reminiscence approaches can enable professionals to take account of the impact of migration, occupation, social and family history in order to make effective assessments and plan appropriate care and therapy. Accurate assessment is important for all older clients, but the social situation of the older people from minority ethnic groups needs sensitive probing if rehabilitation is to be effective. Given the difficulties experienced by some groups, it is essential that rehabilitation and discharge planning take particular note of the difficulties experienced in some communities.

Particular competence is needed to make accurate assessment of cyanosis, anaemia, skin conditions or wound healing in people with dark skin. Pressure-sore risk-assessment tools may be appropriate for the white population but do little to warn of the impending damage to dark skin. Detecting the presence of infection or the extent of wound healing is different in dark skin. The diagnosis and assessment of dementia and depression is complex at the best of times but is complicated by language and the cultural inappropriateness of the tools used (Rait et al 1996,

Richards and Abas 1999). The symptoms of mental illness often coincide with physical problems and a variety of unmet social needs (Richards and Abas 1999) and therefore require cultural knowledge and sensitivity if accurate clinical judgements are to be made.

Clinical skills

A depth of knowledge and clinical expertise is necessary in order to provide good-quality care for all older people, but some additional skill is needed for those from minority ethnic groups (Papadopoulos et al 1998). There are no prescribed protocols, and nurses must learn from patients, carers and particularly colleagues from other cultures (Tilki et al 1994). However, a few specific points relating to the care of older people of African and Caribbean origin merit attention. It is often assumed erro- neously that dark skin is tough and less prone to break, but the reality is to the contrary. The need to oil dark skin regularly may be incongruous with directions to limit the potential for damage caused by rubbing. Nurses must learn when and how to use this essential aspect of the hygiene for patients of African and Caribbean origin. Similarly, nurses need to know how to care for and style the hair of people of African origin. Helping the person to dress requires the practitioner to have some knowledge of how to use a sari or how to fix the headdress worn by African women or the turban for a Sikh man. Relatives will invariably be willing to help demon- strate such skills to nurses and therapists, and practising with the client or on each other can provide opportunities for interaction and even enjoy- ment. Clients, family members or colleagues from particular groups can be asked to contribute to diagrams or other visual aids that highlight the stages involved in helping the client to dress properly.

Engaging the family in identifying, planning, delivering and evaluat- ing culturally appropriate care need not be merely paying lip-service to involvement but can facilitate the fulfilment of their obligations to the older person. Understanding differences in health care beliefs and cultural or religious practices allows for more considered approaches to advice about rehabilitation, treatment or dietary regimens and care.

Therapeutic activities

The importance of activity for older people in residential settings is recog- nized and should be sensitive to the cultural origins of all clients. However, if activities are to be sensitive to the needs of people from minority ethnic groups, they must draw upon relevant cultural informa- tion. Older people from minority ethnic groups are in an ambiguous situation, having psychological links with two societies but perhaps not belonging to either. Reminiscence affords many opportunities to identify cultural issues and to use these to underpin recreational and therapeutic activities. All the functions of reminiscence are appropriate to older people from minority ethnic groups, but, because of their experiences of disadvantage and marginalization, some are more relevant than others (Tilki 2000). Contrary to myths about the extended family, many older people from minority ethnic groups are isolated and alienated (Tilki 1998a, Tilki 1998b). Culturally informed reminiscence can provide enjoyment and social contact in a safe environment and may enhance opportunities to develop friendships and meaningful relationships (Fielden 1990).

Reminiscence activity can be used to keep in touch with the home that older people keep within their hearts. Although the longing to be 'home' is expressed widely as people become older, migration has meant that people become integrated into a global, socio-economic network. The various movements in migratory societies to different parts of the world mean that older people have links which defy national boundaries. In addition to links with home, they may have siblings or children and grandchildren in a number of different countries.

Opportunities for life review are particularly appropriate for older people from minority ethnic groups. Many will grieve for their homeland and families left behind and life review can encourage them to reflect on their current life in a more positive way. They can be encouraged to share unfulfilled hopes, highlight the achievements and acknowledge the courage and determination needed to surmount the obstacles that they faced. They can be helped to recognize the structural forces that led to low income, poor housing and other forms of disadvantage. They can begin to reinterpret what might have been thought of as failure, to value the challenges they have overcome and to prize their achievements and come to terms with their remaining years.

Challenging discrimination

Although the Macpherson Inquiry (1999) relates to the Metropolitan Police Force, it has many implications for nurses and other practitioners. It is no longer acceptable that 'ignorance, unwitting prejudice, thoughtlessness and racist stereotyping' should place at a disadvantage people from minority ethnic groups (Macpherson 1999 p. 321). Nurses have a responsibility to address the gaps in their knowledge and to develop cultural competence in their practice. Equally, there is an onus on organizations to challenge the institutional racism that results in the 'collective failure to provide an appropriate and professional service to people because of their ethnic origin' (Macpherson 1999 p. 321). Nurses and other staff have a crucial role to play in challenging organizational policies, in advising or even demanding action in the interests of their clients.

Valuing diversity

Despite the fact that large numbers of people from different minority ethnic groups work in healthcare, professional training and practice is still largely geared towards the white majority (Gerrish 1999, ALG 2000). Practitioners from different ethnic groups need to feel safe to revisit the values and beliefs of their culture, and to articulate and share them with colleagues in an environment that values and celebrates diversity (Tilki et al 1994). While citizenship, human rights and legislation are logical foundations for good practice, and personal, professional and social enrichment, the delivery of high-quality care and the benefits to the organization might be more motivating.

References

Addington-Hall J (2000) Briefing paper: Care of the dying and the NHS. London: Nuffield Trust.

Askham J, Henshaw L and Tarpey M (1995) Social and health authority services for elderly people from black and minority ethnic communities. London: HMSO.

ALG (Association of London Government) (2000) Sick of being excluded: Improving the health of London's minority ethnic communities. London: Association of London Government.

Aspinall P (1999) Ethnic groups and Our Healthier Nation: Whither the information base? Journal of Public Health Medicine 21 (2): 125–132.

Aspinall P (2000) The challenge of measuring the ethnocultural diversity of Britain in the new millennium. Policy and Politics 28 (1): 109–118.

Bhalla A and Blakemore K (1981) Elders of the minority ethnic groups. Birmingham: AFFOR.

Blakemore K (2000) Health and social care needs in minority communities. Health and Social Care in the Community 8 (1): 22–30.

Blakemore K and Boneham M (1994) Age Race and Ethnicity: A Comparative Approach. Buckingham: Open University Press.

Blaxter M and Patterson E (1982) Mothers and daughters: A three generational study health attitudes and behaviour. Oxford: Heinemann.

Boneham M, Copeland J, Mc Kibbin P, Wilson K, Scott A and Saunders P (1997) Elderly people from ethnic minorities in Liverpool: Mental illness, unmet need and barriers to service use. Health and Social Care in the Community 5 (3): 173–180.

Brownfoot J (1998) The needs of people with dementia and their carers within three ethnic groups in Haringey. London: London Borough of Haringey Housing and Social Services/Alzheimer's Disease Society London Region.

Byron M (1999) The Caribbean-born population in 1990s Britain: Who will return? Journal of Ethnic and Migration Studies 25 (2): 285–301.

Calnan M (1987) Health and illness. London: Tavistock.

Cornwell J (1984) Hard earned lives. London: Tavistock.

Donovan J (1986) We don't buy sickness, it just comes. Aldershot: Gower.

Ebrahim S (1996) Ethnic Elders. British Medical Journal 313: 610–613.

Ebrahim S (1997) Mental health should be measured by the same instrument in different ethnic populations. British Medical Journal 314: 832.

Evandrou M (2000) Social inequalities in Later life: The socio-economic position of older people from ethnic minority ethnic groups in Britain. Population Trends 101: 32–38.

Fielden M (1990) Reminiscence as a therapeutic intervention with sheltered housing residents: A comparative study. British Journal of Social Work 20 (1): 21–24.

Gerrish K (1999) Inequalities in service provision: An examination of institutional influences on the provision of district nursing care to minority ethnic communities. Journal of Advanced Nursing 30 (6): 1263–1271.

Hancock M (1998) Nobody's priority. Open Mind 90 (April) p. 10.

Harding S and Rosato M (1997) Cancer incidence among first generation Scottish, Irish, West Indian and South Asian migrants living in England and Wales. Health Statistics Quarterly 5 pp. 26–27.

Jewson N, Jeffers S and Kalra V S (2000) Older people from Asian Communities in Leicester: A report to Leicester Social Services. Leicester: Leicestershire County Council and University of Leicester.

Johnson M (1976) That was your life: A biographical approach to old age. In: Munnichs J and van den Heuval W (eds) Dependency and interdependency in old age pp. 99–133. The Hague: Martinus Nijhoff.

Jones H (1998) Taking liberties. Open Mind 90 (April): 12–13.

Lowdell C, Evandrou M, Bardsley M, Morgan D and Soljak M (2000) Health of Ethnic Minority Elders in London: Respecting Diversity. London: Health of Londoners Project.

Macpherson W (1999) The Stephen Lawrence Inquiry. Report of an inquiry by Sir William Macpherson of Cluny. London: The Stationery Office.

McCracken C F M, Boneham M A, Copeland J R M, Williams K E, Wilson K, Scott A, McKibben P and Cleave N (1997) Prevalence of dementia and depression among elderly people in Black and ethnic minorities. British Journal of Psychiatry 171 (3): 269–273.

Modood T, Berthoud R, Virdee S, Beishon S, Lakey J (1997) Ethnic Minorities in Britain: diversity and disadvantage. London: Policy Studies Institute.

Nazroo J (1997) The health of Britain's ethnic minorities. London: Policy Studies Institute.

NHSE (1999) National Surveys of NHS patients – General Practice 1998. London: Department of Health.

Papadopoulos I, Tilki M and Taylor I (1998) Transcultural Care: a guide for health care professionals. Salisbury: Quay Books.

Parekh B (2000) The future of multi-ethnic Britain: Report of the Commission on the future of multi-ethnic Britain. London: Runnymede Trust Profile Books.

Patel N (1999) Balanced Enquiry Open Mind July August 1999 pp. 10–11.

Pharoah C (1995) Primary healthcare for elderly people from black and minority ethnic communities. London: HMSO.

Rait G, Burns A and Chew C (1996) Age, ethnicity and mental illness: A triple whammy. British Medical Journal 313 (7069): 1347–8.

Richards M and Abas M (1999) Cross - cultural approaches to dementia and depression in older adults. In: Bhugra D and Bahl V (eds) Ethnicity: An agenda for mental health, Chapter 11 pp. 106–122. London: Gaskell.

Sidell M (1995) Health in old age: Myth, mystery, management. Buckingham: Open University Press.

Smaje C (1995) Health race and ethnicity: Making sense of the evidence. London: Kings Fund Institute.

SSI (Social Services Inspectorate) (1998) They look after their own, don't they? Inspection of community care services for black and older ethnic minority ethnic people. London: Social Services Inspectorate/Department of Health.

Stainton-Rogers W (1991) Explaining health and illness: An exploration of diversity. Hemel Hempstead: Wheatsheaf.

Tilki M, Papadopoulos I, Alleyne J (1994) Learning from colleagues of different cultures. British Journal of Nursing 3 (21): 1118–1124.

Tilki M (1998a) Elderly Irish People in London: A Profile. London: Federation of Irish Societies.

Tilki M (1998b) Old Age in Afro-Caribbean and Asian communities in Britain. In: Papadopoulos I, Tilki M and Taylor G (eds) Transcultural Care: A guide for health professionals pp. 44–68. Salisbury: Quay Books.

Tilki M (2000) Reminiscence. In: Corley G (ed) Older People and Their Needs: A multidisciplinary perspective. London: Whurr.

CHAPTER 12

Health professionals and the older adult

STEPHEN COOK

> 'Growing old is like being increasingly penalized for a crime you haven't committed.'
> Anthony Powell, *Temporary Kings* (1973)

Introduction

During the last quarter of the twentieth century, a number of reports (BMA 1986, Audit Commission 1992, DOH 1994) consistently predicted an increase in the number of older people. In 1986, the British Medical Association predicted a 10 per cent increase in the number of 75-year-olds and a staggering fifty-four per cent increase in the number of 85-year-olds in the population over a twenty-year period (BMA 1986). The Audit Commission (1992) made similar predictions, again suggesting in particular that the numbers of old old (see Chapter 1) would increase significantly.

In addition, the pool of potential informal carers was noted to be falling (Audit Commission 1992). Combined with the implementation of the NHS and Community Care Act (DOH 1990), which placed the responsibility for the assessment of the health and social care needs of older adults on to local authority social services departments, these trends led the Audit Commission to predict an immediate increase in the demand for services from local authorities by older adults (DOH 1990, Audit Commission 1992).

However, recruiting motivated, qualified health professionals to the speciality of care of the older adult has been consistently problematic, especially in nursing (Rands 1972, Bowling and Formby 1991, Murray 1994). Combined with the predictions above, these difficulties have often compromised the ability of service providers to deliver high-quality services for the older adult. This chapter will explore some of the large body of literature and research that has sought to understand and seek solutions to these problems in service provision. It will start by outlining the main explanations offered for the difficulties experienced in recruiting health professionals to the care of the older-adult speciality and, once recruited, retaining them. It will then focus attention on the investigations of the stereotypes and attitudes held by clinicians, educators and students towards older people and their impact on career-pathway choice, job satisfaction and the quality of care. The final part of the chapter will discuss the implications of the research findings for the design of educational programmes preparing individuals for careers in health and social care.

Stereotypes and attitudes

In the British context, several explanations have been offered for the difficulties experienced in recruiting health professionals into the speciality of care of the older adult. They include the late recognition of the care of the older adult as a specialist area of healthcare practice, making it less attractive as a career development option for health professionals. Once identified as a speciality, it acquired low status, possibly because it emerged at a time when the status of older people in British society was declining. For example, it has been suggested that in pre-industrial societies, like Britain in the eighteenth and early nineteenth centuries, old age was associated with a social position that carried both authority and prestige; through property rights, opportunities for continued economic contributions to the community, religious beliefs, family relationships and as repositories of cultural and other useful knowledge, older people acquired authority and influence (Simmons 1945, Simmons 1960 cited in Harris 1990). However, in the nineteenth and twentieth centuries, Britain, like other Western countries, experienced a period of rapid modernization. This collective term incorporates a number of significant social changes, including industrialization (the shift of the workplace from the home or land to the factory) and urbanization (a population shift from rural to urban areas) and the formation of large, corporate organizations with an associated increase in bureaucracy. These changes, it has been argued, were associated with the change in the social position of older people (Silverman 1987). Old age and older people were no longer venerated; they not only lost their authority, but attitudes towards old age and older people in the wider population became increasingly negative and, some would argue, hostile (Love 1988).

More recently, this supposed veneration of older people in earlier times has been questioned and, in some cases, challenged as a myth (Wright 1998). However, most authors agree that, throughout the twentieth century, attitudes towards old age and older people among the wider population did change and Elder (1977) and Phillipson (1982) argue that these negative attitudes were responsible for the increased isolation and alienation of older adults as a social group.

In the process, old age and older people acquired a negative stereotype, which they carried with them into the healthcare context, where 'geriatrics', and geriatric nursing in particular, acquired the image of a 'low-tech Cinderella service' (Wright 1998 p. 4). Consequently, 'geriatric patients' came to share a marginalized status with other client groups similarly adversely stigmatized by negative stereotypes and attitudes, such as people with a mental illness and those with a learning disability, making the specialities associated with these client groups less attractive to work in (see Chapter 9).

Recruiting and retaining staff

Explanations offered for the difficulties experienced in retaining health professionals once recruited to the care of the older-adult speciality include the stress associated with the work derived from the particular configuration of 'stressors' involved in caring for the older adult:

- the interpersonal tensions and emotional demands involved in caring for clients with enduring and incurable health problems,
- tensions inside the work group, including interprofessional conflict over the most appropriate interventions to be employed in patient care,
- forces outside the work group, such as insufficient resources,
- unrealistic self-expectations, an all-pervasive stressor because they have their roots in the value and belief systems, and the associated socialization processes, operating within the healthcare professions and their training programmes: 'Helpers give help in certain prescribed ways, with certain expected outcomes ... When the helper cannot feel helpful in an expected or desired way, the result is stress' (Scully 1983 p. 193).

The potential consequences of the stressor configurations experienced by people working with the vulnerable older adult were starkly revealed by the publication of eyewitness accounts of the horrific treatment, including physical and psychological neglect and actual cruelty, of institutionalized older patients (Robb 1967). Stannard (1973) found similar neglect and cruelty in the care of the older adult in his study in the United States. Together, these two reports led to numerous urgent investigations into the care of the older adult, many of them focusing on nursing care. Ingham and Fielding suggest that these early investigations saw attitudes as the key to the problem: 'Attitudes were seen to be defective and in some way responsible for the unsatisfactory treatment of patients' (Ingham and Fielding 1985). The author's own experiences of both caring for older adults and organizing, delivering and supervising students undertaking care-of-the-older-adult components of professional educational programmes suggest that the issue of attitudes remains significant, but perhaps in a rather more complex way than was first assumed.

Studies of attitudes and their relationship to behaviours

The majority of studies investigating attitudes towards older people among health professionals have tended to focus on students, unqualified and qualified personnel, or a combination of all three; generally, they have tended to demonstrate negative attitudes (e.g. Tatham 1982). Even where positive attitudes have been identified, they have not reflected a desire to work with the older adult after qualification (Astrom 1986, Fielding 1986). This suggests that educational strategies fail to generate a sustainable interest and intention to work with older people after qualification (Astrom 1986) and, consequently, recruitment to this speciality remains problematic.

This work, however, has proved to be problematic for a number of reasons:

- theoretically, because the studies assume a direct relationship between attitudes and observable behaviour
- methodologically, because quantitative methods dominate the investigations of this subject
- because findings from various studies often conflict with one another.

Each of these problems, and their associated literature, will be discussed in turn.

Not surprisingly, there are conceptual and theoretical problems involved in the study of attitudes. For example, McGuire (1985) highlights the problems researchers have had in defining the concept 'attitude'. He suggests this is partly due to the term having acquired specialist and lay meanings. To illustrate this point, he cites the Azjen and Fishbein (1977) review of two hundred studies (McGuire 1985) in which seventy per cent of them defined attitudes in more than one way, yielding more than five hundred operational definitions. This conceptual diversity makes comparisons between studies difficult and raises important doubts about the theoretical frameworks developed from them.

In addition, different disciplines tend to conceptualize attitudes differently. For example, psychologists tend to work with operational definitions of attitudes that delineate them as 'enduring cognitive evaluations' (Rathus 1990 p. 601). Sociologists and social psychologists, however, tend to work with a model of attitudes that incorporates affective (i.e. feelings), behavioural and cognitive elements (Breckler 1984), attitudes becoming an expression of the interaction between these three domains.

Inconsistencies

A major theoretical issue relates to the ability of attitudes to explain or predict observed behaviour. Numerous researchers have questioned the correlation between attitudes and observed behaviour (Azjen and Fishbein 1977, Cialdini et al 1981), and, as Coon points out, 'there are often large differences between attitudes and behaviour – particularly between privately held attitudes and public behaviour' (Coon 1989 p. 647). For example, Fishbein and Azjen (1975) suggest that individuals can actually hold a negative set of attitudes towards an object, person or group (e.g. old people) but still behave positively towards them. Also, great pressure to conform to undesirable institutional norms may provoke negative behaviours in staff with positive attitudes.

Investigations of the relationship between identified attitudes and behaviour suggest there are several important factors influencing the behavioural expression of attitudes:

- the *specificity* of an attitude, i.e. very specific attitudes are more reliable predictors of behaviour than more global ones: 'We can better predict church attendance by knowing people's attitudes towards the importance of regular church attendance than by knowing more globally whether they are Christian' (Rathus 1990 p. 601)
- the *strength* of an attitude; strongly held attitudes provide more reliable explanations or predictions of behaviour than weakly held attitudes (Rathus 1990 p. 601)

- the *vested interest* dimension; individuals are more likely to act, or behave, in accordance with an attitude if they have a vested interest in the outcome of its expression (Rathus 1990 p. 602).

While other factors may affect the expression of an attitude in behavioural terms, those identified above are particularly pertinent to studies conducted into nurses' attitudes towards older people. Although some authors have concluded that there *is* a positive correlation between positive attitudes and high-quality nursing care (e.g. LaMonica 1979), the studies on which these conclusions are based have only measured the positive or negative quality of the attitudes, ignoring their specificity, strength or any vested interests that might be operating in their behavioural expression. Kayser and Menningerode (1975) suggest that nursing students and other healthcare providers with stereotyped attitudes towards older people are more likely to prefer working with older patients, which poses particular problems for recruitment strategies and suggests a need for caution in drawing any conclusions about the relationship between attitudes and the quality of care.

Despite the failure to demonstrate conclusively a direct correlation between attitudes and behaviour, Ingham and Fielding (1985) still argue the importance of studying nurses' behaviour and the factors that affect it, including attitudes, in an attempt to improve the provision of care. Such an assertion would seem reasonable only if the field of investigation was widened both theoretically and methodologically, to take into account the complex picture emerging from the above discussion. For example, the majority of studies investigating students' and qualified nurses' attitudes towards older people have adopted the theoretical framework that assumes a correlation between measured attitudes and observable behaviour. Consequently, the methods adopted have tended to rely on quantitative data collected through attitude questionnaires, knowledge-based questionnaires or a combination of both (Ingham and Fielding 1985) focused on quantifying negative- and positive-attitude orientations in their subjects to compare with the quality of care. Single-attitude studies have been by far the most common.

However, the use of attitude-measurement tools has not been consistent, making comparisons between studies difficult (Ingham and Fielding 1985). Although most of the questionnaires used have been validated to some extent by repeated use, they all tend to treat attitudes as one-dimensional (see above). This theoretical weakness is reflected in the methodologies adopted, which have been quantitative and narrow in focus, largely ignoring the interactive and contextual elements affecting their formation, expression and maintenance or change of attitudes, and organizational influences on behaviour.

However, some studies have attempted to identify the attitudes of their subjects without using attitude scales, but have still adopted a quantitative approach to data collection and analysis. For example, Armstrong-Esther et al (1989) used observational techniques to measure the quantity of time spent by nurses in interacting with older-adult clients, and then determined the quality of this time by noting the type of interaction taking place within it. Conversational interaction denoted 'high quality' time, while interaction consisting predominantly of statements by staff, usually instructions, denoted low-quality interaction. While an interesting way of gaining access to, and drawing inferences about, attitudes, and their relationship to the quality of care, the study still assumes that positive behaviours are expressions of positive attitudes. In another study, Giardina-Roche and Black (1989) use the person-perception paradigm for measuring attitudes towards the older adult among students.

Another major problem with these studies is their use of the concepts of positive and negative attitudes; rarely is there any discussion about how attitudes are so classified or whether these perceptions of positivity and negativity of attitudes are shared by their subjects. In short, the pursuit of meaningful quantitative data has been compromised by the adoption of methodologies that fail to take account, or control, of other important variables that may be influencing the behavioural expression of attitudes.

While interesting as methods for accessing attitudes, neither these nor previous studies attempted to measure changes in attitudes following educational interventions, or examine their relationship to a future-career choice. Studies investigating the impact of educational interventions on students' attitudes towards the older adult have a long history. Thirty years ago, Evans (1969) showed that common stereotypes and negative attitudes associated with the older adult could be changed in student nurses if they experienced healthy older adults living independently prior to their exposure to the dependent older adult in receipt of healthcare. Hart et al (1976) and Brock (1977) obtained similar results. However, Greenhill and Baker (1986) found no significant difference in the level of knowledge about, or positive attitudes towards, older adults between two groups of students, the first exposed to healthy older adults before their exposure to the older adult in clinical settings, and another group not so exposed.

Fielding (1979) demonstrates that nurses' attitudes towards older adult clients were not uniform across different settings. She found older adult

clients in continuing-care settings were rated significantly more negatively than older adult clients receiving outpatient hospital care.

Psychological studies demonstrating a revision of stereotypes and attitudes in the face of new information (Weber and Crocker 1983) have been
supported by studies exploring the impact of new information and knowledge about the ageing process on student nurses' attitudes towards the
older adult. Ross (1983) demonstrates that an increase in knowledge was
associated with a revision of negative attitudes among student nurses, and
Quinn-Krach and Van Hoozer (1988) demonstrate not only a positive
correlation between the level of knowledge in students and favourable
attitudes towards older adults but also higher levels of knowledge and
more positive attitudes among older students. Interestingly, but not
surprisingly, they also demonstrated a relationship between ethnicity,
levels of knowledge and attitudes, suggesting that various cultural variables may be operating in the behavioural expression of attitudes.

Although measuring changes in attitudes following different educational
interventions is interesting, it is more important to know whether positive
changes are sustained over time and whether they influence students in their
career choices after qualification. While a shift of attitudes in a positive
direction following educational interventions may be desirable, it will not
necessarily generate the supply of motivated, high-calibre staff required in
this area of healthcare unless positive attitudes towards older adults are the
only determining factor in the future-career choices of students.

Attitudes and career choice – two key studies

Two studies that did focus on the relationship between attitudes and
future-career choice were Astrom (1986) and Fielding (1986). Astrom's
study measured the intentions of 315 final-year nursing students in
Sweden to work with clients suffering from dementias before and after a
care-of-the-older-adult module in an education programme. Unfortunately, it is limited for two reasons. First, because it focused only on the
intention to work with clients with a dementing illness, limiting its potential for more universal application. Second, because it is impossible to
know whether the perceived change was due to the educational input or
some other variable. Nevertheless, its recognition that older clients suffering from a particular condition may be more unpopular than others is
important, because clients suffering from a dementia constitute a large
proportion of older adults requiring continuing care.

Fielding (1986) argues that it is a mistake to see specific educational interventions, such as care of the older-adult modules, in isolation from the rest of

a training programme. Her student-nurse subjects showed a decreasing desire to work in the care-of-the-older-adult speciality as they went through their course, irrespective of any positive shift in attitudes towards older adults, and whether or not they enjoyed care-of-the-older-adult placements. A third of her sample at the end of their course described the older-adult speciality as boring and physically taxing, and lacking the type of experiences useful to career progression. Consequently, only ten per cent were considering working in the older-adult speciality after completing their course.

Pre-course influences

Findings relating to pre-course experiences of older adults seem equally conflicting. Giardina-Roche and Black (1989) found that students who had close relationships with their grandparents held more positive attitudes towards older adults. However, Hart et al (1976) found that first-year baccalaureate nursing students who had worked with older adults had significantly poorer attitudes than students without such experience. If student nurses have no pre-course experiences with older adults, often their first encounter with them is with those experiencing health or social difficulties requiring some sort of intervention by professionals. Many may be highly dependent, confused and difficult to communicate with, or have low levels of arousal, episodes of incontinence or aggressive tendencies. Some may present all of these features and require an intense level of care, demanding complex skills to deliver care effectively; skills that are frequently underestimated and undervalued, even in the course curricula for health professionals, reinforcing a detrimental impact on the development of positive attitudes towards older adults (Langland et al 1986), and decreasing the likelihood of health professionals selecting the care of the older adult as a post-qualifying speciality-career choice (Gunter 1973, Kayser and Menningerode 1975, Chamberland et al 1978).

Changing attitudes

Most educational interventions in nursing courses adopt the framework conceived by Triandis (1971) for changing attitudes and stereotypes relating to older adults in a positive direction. The framework includes:

- provision of new information
- provision of experiences in the presence of the attitude subject
- forcing a person to act (i.e. once an event has taken place, attitudes change to become consistent with the new event).

However, four other important factors may influence the formation of students' attitudes towards the care of the older adult:

- views and attitudes of contemporary society towards older adults and ageing
- the individual student's previous experience of older adults
- views and attitudes of the teaching staff
- attitudes of trained health professionals (Tatham 1982).

Clearly, the potential for educational interventions to overcome all four influences is severely limited and should caution all concerned from viewing educational interventions as the universal panacea for the problem.

Implications of research findings

While the issues discussed above make direct comparison between studies problematic, it is notable that many of the published findings appear to conflict with one another. Nevertheless, they do provide some insight into those areas that might be relevant to all those involved in the care of the older adult, be it as clinician, service manager or educationalist. They also point to those areas requiring further detailed investigation, particularly in relation to career pathway choice. Ingham and Fielding (1986) suggest that future research should attempt to avoid the proliferation of ambiguous studies using questionable techniques by addressing the *real* issues in a careful and meaningful way. Unfortunately, they failed to identify what they considered to be the *real* issues, or the techniques they considered appropriate for investigating them. A hint of what they *might* have meant can be derived from the report of a study conducted by Fielding, where she argues that, while: 'the concept of "attitude" has been used to predict behaviour, [it] has not been able to answer the more interesting and vital question – why? Neither simple attitudinal measurements, nor simple behavioural measurements can offer an explanation,'(Fielding 1986 p. 30).

In order to address this problem, she adopted a methodology for her study grounded in the philosophical and theoretical perspectives of 'new paradigm research' (Reason and Rowan 1981), and, in particular, a theory of action outlined by Harré as: '[the belief] that people are agents acting intentionally in accordance with socially grounded rules and conventions to realize projects' (Harré 1981 p. 16).

This theoretical perspective makes the focus of Fielding's empirical investigation quite different from the majority of studies conducted in this

area. Instead of investigating the (dubious!) relationship between an attitude measured in one situation (with questionable measuring instruments) and an overt behaviour in a different context, she focuses on
identifying, and capitalizing on 'the intentions and meanings people give
to their actions. The identification of meaning is seen to be at the heart of
the explanation of behaviour' (Fielding 1986 p. 30). This approach does
not preclude a quantitative approach, but it opens up the field of investigation to qualitative methods, or a combination of the two. As Harré
(1981) points out: 'As a positivist, one is counselled to study the confidence levels of correlations between types of treatments and types of
effects through examining numbers of cases. By adopting this advice, one
can avoid the deep study of the internal processes and activities of agents
which bring these effects about.' (Harré 1981 p. 14.)

According to Fielding (1986), this explains the failure of research in
this area to make any headway, or answer the questions it sets out to,
because it employs a methodology that assumes that what people say or
do can be studied in isolation from social context and outside the meanings employed by participants, denying them the possibility of 'human'
responses.

Interestingly, research in this area declined in the 1990s, a trend possibly influenced by some of the complexities surrounding the research of
attitudes and their influence on behaviour and career choice. However, it
is a trend more likely to have been influenced by the enactment of the
NHS and community-care legislation (DoH 1990) at the beginning of the
1990s, which led to a shift in the provision of care for the older adult from
institutional to community settings. This shift, inevitably, led to a greater
reliance on families, relatives and neighbours for the delivery of care to
dependent older adults. Not surprisingly, lay carers were as equally, if not
more, vulnerable as health and social care professionals to becoming
overwhelmed by the responsibilities and emotional demands engendered
in caring for a dependent older adult. Increasing financial constraints in
the public services, making the provision of support for lay carers even
more problematic, compounded such 'burdens' of care. It is hardly
surprising, therefore, that lay carers faced with similar, if not greater,
levels of stress than those experienced by professionals providing care in
institutional settings in the 1960s and 1970s became susceptible to the
perpetration of abuse against their frail older relatives. As increasing
numbers of such cases became known to health and social care professionals working in the primary sectors, so the focus of research, under-
standably, shifted to the plight of lay carers (Pritchard 1992).

Developing positive attitudes

Given the demographic trends identified in this and other chapters, an increased demand for health and social services from the growing older population may indeed materialize and must be taken seriously. However, it must be considered in the wider context, which involves the recognition that old age does not necessarily lead to increasing infirmity and demand for care. Even before the drive towards community care, ninety-five per cent of older adults requiring care received it from relatives in their own homes, or in the homes of their relatives, demanding little from health and social services (BMA 1986). Also, studies in Canada have suggested that it is often a minority of the older adult population that accounts for a disproportionate level of health and social service utilization (Victor 1987).

Nevertheless, if the predicted increase in demand for health and social services from an increasingly older population materializes, there will be an even greater need to attract newly qualifying professionals to work with this client group and their lay carers. Hence, there is still an urgent need for greater insight into the factors that make recruitment and retention of staff to this area of practice problematic. Simply asserting that, 'Elderly care now offers dynamic career opportunities' (Factfile 1989 p. 569) has not made the problem go away. Nor has shifting the locus of care delivery from institutional to community settings necessarily led to an improved quality of care or life for older adults. Twenty years ago, Brower suggested there was an urgent need to investigate the impact of social organization on the attitudes of health professionals, including nurses, towards the older adult, because: 'a reciprocal relationship develops, in which the organization and actors (nurses) influence each other ... The social group of the organization serves as a significant other in inculcating abilities, values, and perceptions' (Brower 1981 p. 294).

In other words, behaviour is influenced just as much, if not more, by external as opposed to internal factors, such as attitudes, values and beliefs (Salmon 1993). Consequently, students are just as likely to interpret the behaviour of older adults, qualified professional staff or organizations as manifestations of the attitudes held by those groups about students. This means that educational interventions alone are highly unlikely to create or sustain positive attitudes towards the older adult in students or to influence their decisions whether or not to work in the care-of-the-older-adult speciality on qualification. However, by changing the educational focus on to preparing students for the 'gap' between theory and practice, which appears from the literature to be particularly acute in care-of-the-older-adult settings, it may be possible to reduce the level of anxiety experienced by students and facilitate an exploration of the socio-logical, psychological and organizational forces generating the situations they encounter in the care-of-the-older-adult placements.

Conclusions

After reviewing the literature, one is left with the feeling that the solutions to the problems associated with the care of older adults have been identi-fied; however, these solutions may be so radical that they threaten too many vested interests. In a move to improve standards for older clients in need of long-term care, the Abbots Langley hospital established a unit that dispensed with qualified nursing staff because they were perceived as part of, rather than a solution to, the problem (Brindle 1990). If this view is correct, a more fundamental reassessment of the attitudes, values and belief systems operating in healthcare occupations is surely called for, together with an assessment of the role played by educationalists and healthcare organizations in propagating them.

To anyone who experienced the working conditions of health profes-sionals, especially nurses, under which the abuse of older adults was perpetrated in the 1960s and 1970s, it is clear that those professionals were themselves the victims of abuse by organizations and governments who failed to provide them with the resources needed to provide the health and social care required by the older adults in their charge. In the same way, today's lay carers are the potential victims of abuse by a system that fails to provide them with the physical resources and psychological support they need to care for their older relatives. How to break this cycle of abuse is perhaps the most challenging subject for anyone involved in the care of older adults today.

References.

Armstrong-Esther C A, Sandilands M L and Miller D (1989) Attitudes and behaviours of nurses towards the elderly in an acute care setting. Journal of Advanced Nursing 14 (1): 34–41.

Astrom S (1986) Healthcare students' attitudes towards, and intention to work with, patients suffering from senile dementia. Journal of Advanced Nursing 11 (6): 651–659.

Audit Commission for Local Authorities and the National Health Service for England and Wales (1992) Community Care: Managing the Cascade of Change, NHS Report 6. London: HMSO.

Azjen I and Fishbein M (1977) Attitude-Behaviour relations: A theoretical analysis and review of empirical research. Psychological Bulletin 84: 888–918.

Bowling A and Formby J (1991) Nurses' attitudes to elderly people: a survey of nursing homes and elderly care wards in an Inner-London health district. Nursing Practice 5 (1): 16–24.

Breckler S J (1984) Empirical validation of affect, behavior, and cognition as distinct components of attitude. Journal of Personality and Social Psychology 47: 1191–1205.

Brindle D (1990) A happy ward with no nurses. The Guardian Friday 14 September.

British Medical Association (1986) All our tomorrows: Growing old in Britain. London: BMA Board of Science and Education.

Brock A M (1977) Improving Nursing Care for the elderly: An educational task. Journal of Gerontological Nursing 3 (1): 26–28.

Brower H T (1981) Social Organization and Nurses' Attitudes Toward Older Persons. Journal of Gerontological Nursing 7 (5): 293–298.

Chamberland G, Rawls B, Powell C and Roberts M J (1978) Improving students' attitudes toward aging. Journal of Gerontological Nursing 4 (1): 44–45.

Cialdini R B, Petty R E and Cacippo T J (1981) Attitude and attitude change. Annual Review of Psychology 32: 357–404.

Coon D (1989) Introduction to Psychology: Exploration and Application 6th edn. St Paul: West Publishing Co.

DOH (Department of Health) (1990) NHS & Community Care Act. London: HMSO.

DOH (Department of Health) (1994) Social Trends 24. London: HMSO.

Elder G (1977) The Alienated: Growing Old Today. London: Writers and Readers Publishing Co-operative.

Evans F M C (1969) Visiting older people: A learning experience. Nursing Outlook 17 (March): 20–22.

Factfile (1989) Elderly care now offers dynamic career opportunities. Professional Nurse 4 (11): 569–570.

Fielding P (1979) An exploratory investigation of self-concept in the institutionalized elderly, and a comparison with nurses' conceptions and attitudes. International Journal of Nursing Studies 16: 345–354

Fielding P (1986) Attitudes Revisited: An Examination of Student Nurses' Attitudes Towards Old People in Hospital. London: Royal College of Nursing.

Fishbein M and Azjen I (1975) Belief, Attitude, Intention and Behaviour: An Introduction to Theory and Research. Reading, Mass: Addison-Wesley.

Giardina-Roche C and Black (1989) Attitudes of diploma student nurses toward adult clients. Journal of Nursing Education 29 (5): 208–214.

Greenhill E D and Baker M R (1986) The effects of a well older adult clinical experience on students' knowledge and attitudes. Journal of Nurse Education 25 (4): 145–147.

Gunter C M (1973) Attitudes of nursing personnel toward the aged. Nursing Research 22: 517–520.

Harré R (1981) The positivist-empiricist approach and its alternative. In: Reason P and Rowan I (eds) Human Inquiry: A Sourcebook of New Paradigm Research pp. 3–17. Chichester: John Wiley and Sons.

Harris D K (1990) Sociology of Aging, 2nd edn. London: Harper and Row.

Hart L K, Freed M I and Cromwell C M (1976) Changing attitudes toward the aged and interest in caring for the aged. Journal of Gerontological Nursing 2 (1): ll–16.

Ingham R and Fielding P (1985) A review of nursing literature on attitudes towards old people. International Journal of Nursing Studies 22 (3): 171–181.

Kayser J S and Menningerode F A (1975) Increasing nursing students' interest in working with aged patients. Nursing Research 24: 23–26.

LaMonica E L (1979) The nurse and the ageing client: positive attitude formation Nurse Educator 4: 23–26

Langland R M, Raithel J, Benjamin B, Crim B and Kunz C (1986) Change in basic nursing students' attitudes toward the elderly after a nursing home experience. Journal of Nursing Education 25 (1): 31–33.

Love C (1988) Applying the Nursing Process with the Elderly. In: Wilson H and Kneisl C (eds) Psychiatric Nursing 3rd edn. Wokingham: Adison-Wesley.

McGuire W J (1985) Attitudes and attitude change In Lindsey G and Aronson E (eds) Handbook of Social Psychology 3rd edn. 2: 233–346. New York: Random House.

Murray K (1994) Personal Communication from Senior Nurse Manager, Whittington Hospital, London (unpublished).

Phillipson C (1982) Capitalism and the Construction of Old Age. London: Macmillan.

Pritchard J (1992) The Abuse of Elderly People: A Handbook for Professionals. London: Jessica Kingsley Publishers.

Quinn-Krach P and Van Hoozer H (1988) Sexuality of the aged and the attitudes and knowledge of nursing students. Journal of Nurse Education. 27 (8): 359–363.

Rands V H (1972) Geriatric Nursing Services. Nursing Times 68: 1054–1057.

Rathus S A (1990) Psychology. Orlando: Holt, Rinehart & Winston.

Reason P and Rowan J (eds) (1981) Human Inquiry: A Sourcebook of New Paradigm Research. Chichester: John Wiley and Sons.

Robb B (1967) Sans Everything: A Case to Answer. London: Nelson.

Ross M M (1983) Learning to nurse the elderly: outcome measures. Journal of Advanced Nursing 8: 373–378.

Salmon P (1993) Interactions of nurses with elderly patients: relationship to nurses' attitudes and to formal activity periods. Journal of Advanced Nursing 18 (1): 14–19.

Scully R (1983) The Work-Setting Support Group: A Means of Preventing Burnout. In: Farber B (ed) Stress and Burnout in the Human Service Professions. Oxford: Pergamon Press.

Silverman P (1987) Family Life. In: Silverman P (ed) The Elderly as Pioneers pp. 205–223 Bloomington: Indiana University Press.

Simmons L W (1945) The Role of the Aged in Primitive Society. New Haven: Yale University Press.

Simmons L W (1960) Aging in preindustrial societies. In: Toward Better Understanding of the Aging pp. 1–8. New York: Council on Social Work Education.

Stannard C I (1973) Old folks and dirty work: The social conditions for patient abuse in a nursing home. Social Problems 20: 329–342.

Tatham S A (1982) Factors which influence learners attitudes to the elderly. British Journal of Geriatric Nursing 12–13.

Triandis H C (1971) Attitudes and Attitude Change. Toronto: John Wiley.

Victor C R (1987) Old Age in Modern Society. London: Chapman & Hall.

Weber R and Crocker J (1983) Cognitive processes in the revision of stereotypic beliefs. Journal of Personality and Social Psychology 45: 961–977.

Wright SG (1998) Introduction. In: Marr J and Kershaw B (eds) Caring for Older People: Developing specialist practice pp. 1–9. London: Arnold.

CHAPTER 13

The older adult in the mass media

STEPHEN COOK

Introduction

On Monday 20 November 2000, Victor Meldrew died. You may have been one of the many millions of British television viewers who mourned his death, because he had been the principal character in one of the BBC's most successful situation comedies, *One Foot in the Grave*. Starting in 1990, for ten years the series charted the trials and tribulations of a retired 'older adult' coming to terms with increasing age and frequently greeting a rapidly changing world with the exclamation, '*I don't believe it!*'

Why should we be interested in how 'older adults' are portrayed on television? Or in the other mass media, such as films, radio, magazines and newspapers? The short answer to these questions is that, while some of the myths and stereotypes commonly associated with 'old age' may not have originated in the mass media, there is still a common belief that the mass media are responsible for disseminating and perpetuating them (Harris, 1990). This is hardly surprising, given that ever since the invention of the printing press, books, periodicals, magazines and newspapers have been, and still are, seen by governments, pressure groups and other social institutions as a means of influencing the thoughts, values, beliefs and behaviours of those exposed to them or, as McQuail (2000) suggests, as sources of power that can be mobilized to control, manage or otherwise influence society – an effective alternative to the use of force.

Add to the printed media the development of radio, film and television, and their capability for communicating messages to large numbers of individuals simultaneously as collective, amorphous (mass) audiences, it's not surprising that researchers have chosen to investigate the validity of the claims that the mass media are instrumental in the formation, production, dissemination and maintenance or change of stereotypes and attitudes in their audiences.

In addition, the twentieth century was the period that saw the mass media emerge as enormous institutions, with their own rules, norms and links to society and other social institutions, like governments. In the process, they became major providers of employment, goods and services, another dimension to their activity meriting systematic study in the fields of social psychology, sociology and the newly created discipline of media studies (McQuail 2000).

As television is still perceived by many to be the most powerful purveyor of images and stereotypes (Victor 1987, Harris 1990), the first part of this chapter will continue the focus on the portrayal of the older adult in this medium. It will then widen its scope by looking at the findings of those (relatively few) studies that have explored the portrayal of 'older adults' in the mass media more generally. Of much more interest to students of the media, however, is the extent to which their messages or representations have an impact on, or influence, the values, beliefs and behaviours of their audiences. In this domain, we are forced to rely on the numerous studies of the impact of media representations of sex and violence on audiences' beliefs and behaviours. While the extent to which such studies can help us understand the impact of media representations of 'older adults' on their audiences is debatable, the theoretical frameworks such studies have generated are nevertheless of relevance, especially when we come to consider future research into the impact of media representations of older adults. Therefore, subsequent parts of the chapter will explore the relevance of the findings and theories emerging from media studies more generally to our understanding of media representations of older adults and their implications for health care service providers and professionals.

The case of the television situation comedy

Returning to the television situation comedy, it could be argued that, although much loved by the many millions of viewers who regularly switched on to watch and laugh at the hilarious situations he encountered, the character of Victor Meldrew nevertheless encapsulated a common stereotype of the older adult: forgetful, slow to catch on to what was happening and hence open to misunderstanding, rigid, and suspicious of change. However, many of the more bizarre situations he experienced resulted from his refusal to allow what he perceived, quite rightly, as disrespectful treatment of the 'older adult' by others to go unchallenged. But such a stance, while not portrayed as foolish, was nevertheless portrayed as eccentric, and perceived as such by both his wife and neighbours, who found his refusal to accept the status quo as exasperating.

During the same ten-year period, another equally successful British television situation comedy, *Waiting for God*, generated humour from the joint rebellions of two 'older adults', Diana and Tom, against the attempts of their children and other people in authority to get them to conform to the attitudes and behaviours considered appropriate for people 'their age'. Although Diana and Tom were given the attributes of vitality, boldness of character, courage, determination, rebelliousness, mischievousness and sexuality, the action of the series took place against the backdrop of the Bay View Retirement Home, where the other residents invariably displayed a host of the less-desirable attributes commonly associated with old age, (listlessness, detachment, stupidity, resignation and disorientation), thus creating the impression that Tom and Diana were the exceptions rather than the rule.

For those unfamiliar with British television, the two series referred to above represent the latest in a line of situation comedies revolving around the characters of 'older adults' that spanned the latter half of the twentieth century. It could be argued that, although these two series, as a whole, upheld the negative stereotypes associated with old age, they nevertheless portrayed older adulthood far more favourably and sympathetically than two of their equally famous and successful predecessors: *'Till Death Us Do Part* and *Steptoe and Son*. These two situation comedies ran through the 1960s and 1970s, and in both the central older-adult characters were far from attractive and endearing. In *'Till Death Us Do Part*, Alf Garnett, both the lead character and an 'older adult', was portrayed as a bigoted, racist and misogynist character, while, in *Steptoe and Son*, Harold Steptoe's elderly father was portrayed as withered, toothless and lecherous, and was frequently addressed by his own son as 'you dirty old man'.

Earlier media studies

In 1983 (Lambert 1984), a team of fourteen people aged between 33 and 73 years was used to evaluate both the frequency with which older adults appeared, and the way in which they were portrayed, in all television programmes transmitted on four British television channels during a two-week period in the winter of 1983. The programmes included drama, light entertainment, current affairs and news transmissions. For the purpose of the study, 'older adult' was defined as anyone over the age of 60.

Overall, the study found that older adults appeared in 62% of BBC 1, 51% of BBC 2, 57 % of ITV and 63% of Channel 4 transmissions; all relatively high percentages given the numbers of older adults in the general population. However, closer analysis revealed that:

- most of the older adults who made up these high percentages were appearing in current affairs, documentary and news programmes
- the majority of them were 'world leaders': politicians, diplomats and other dignitaries
- the vast majority of these 'older adults' were males.

In addition, when current affairs programmes were excluded from the analysis:

- the percentage of older adults dropped considerably
- when older adults did appear in drama serials, soap operas, children's and adventure programmes, they tended to be peripheral rather than central characters
- although generally portrayed as fit and healthy, their sexuality was frequently played down, as were the financial hardships frequently experienced by older adults in the wider community
- television programmes tended to distinguish between the 'young' and 'old' older age person (interestingly, a distinction now commonly made in the study of older adults and in the health care context)
- the 'young older age' were nearly always portrayed as more active and assertive than the 'old older age'
- the 'old older age' were least likely to appear in television programmes
- despite their numerical dominance, older women were significantly underrepresented in television programmes.

The overall implications of the study were that the older older adult tends to be invisible as far as television is concerned and that the representations of older adults overall tend to incline towards negative stereotypes.

Gender perspectives

The study also supported much earlier observations of what Sontag (1978) refers to as the 'double standard', and Itzin (1984) as the 'double jeopardy', of ageing applied to women in the media; where women in the media were concerned, they had to contend with ageism compounded with sexism. The awareness of this 'double standard' emerged with the women's movement in the late 1960s. While it originally focused on the portrayal of younger women, it eventually incorporated the plight of older women as well who, it was observed, were generally portrayed as weak and helpless, and constantly exhorted by the media to stay young and beautiful or to disguise their true age (Victor 1987). In other words, the media helped to reinforce the notion that women should live up to a youthful ideal throughout their lives in a way that men need not; a situation that seems to have remained much the same over the years because, in 1993, nearly fifteen years after Sontag's and Itzin's observations, Susan Moore is led to pose the questions:

> Do John Simpson or Jon Snow or Peter Sissons worry about their lines, their paunches or their greying hair? Do their editors feel these old boys should not be inflicted on the rest of us any longer? Do we worry about the emptiness of their private lives as we seem to do with [Kate] Adie? (Moore 1993).

Prime-time television

Another dimension to television representations of older adults relates to what is called 'prime-time' television; the period between 20:00 and 23:00 hours when a third of all television viewing takes place. Interestingly, older adults are markedly underrepresented on prime-time television, and, when they do appear, they are more likely to be cast in minor roles and to be seen being treated more disrespectfully than those in any other age group (Harris 1990).

If the focus on the humorous representations of old age and the older adult is widened to include cartoons in newspapers and magazines, on greetings cards, in jokes told by stand-up comedians and comedy sketches in television light-entertainment shows, again we find a strong inclination towards negative stereotyping of the older adult and the ageing process. For example, Palmore (1971, 1986) analyses the content of jokes, cartoons and greeting cards about ageing and finds that over half portray highly negative, and in some cases openly hostile, attitudes towards the older adult. A number of themes emerge relating to the butt of the humour: longevity, physical, sexual and/or mental abilities and age concealment, the humour frequently reflecting 'common-sense' observations and glib generalizations.

Recent studies

Interesting as these content-analysis studies of media representations of older adults and the ageing process are, more recent media research suggests that the situation is far more complex. Rrbye (1995), for example, in a study of Danish national and local newspaper articles appearing in 1994, relating to the older adult conducts a multi-level analysis of the material informed by critical and post-modern theories of language, communication and narration and found that:

- one article may contain several and very different images of old age
- articles often form part of a 'media drama' which can run over a long period of time
- the prejudicial effects of the mass media may be more influenced by the receivers' existing images and attitudes.

Similarly, Warnes (1995) suggests that representations of old age and the older adults in both the media and policy discourse are unstable, frequently swinging from one dominant stereotype to another, making systematic comparisons of cultural and media representations of old age and the older adult methodologically complex.

For example, a content analysis of the portrayal of over 14,000 television characters on American television between 1969 and 1981 (Signorelli 1989) found that:

- while the very old were under-represented in prime-time television drama, this was also true for the very young
- although older characters were more likely to be portrayed as 'bad', they were less likely to be involved in violence than younger characters
- while 70% of older men and 80% of older women were portrayed as low status, and treated disrespectfully, such representations were still patchy

In a review of studies exploring age stereotyping in the media, Biggs (1993) suggests that although a more positive and active image of ageing could be discerned in British television, the picture was still complex. For example:

- while situation comedies often contain 'reverse stereotyping' of the older adult, they are often portrayed as unrealistic exceptions; far more common is the portrayal of older people as feeble, vague, forgetful and cantankerous
- while soap operas tend to be dominated by the middle-aged and older adults, there is often a lack of focus on the problems of age and ageing, and discrepancies in the images of men and women; for example, Dail (1988) found that soap operas were more likely to portray older women in a positive way.

These discrepancies are not restricted to television either; Featherstone and Wernick (1995), for example, have pointed out the preponderance of older men in radio programmes such as *Gardeners' Question Time* and *Just a Minute*, although there is evidence that this is changing.

The diverse, and often contradictory, findings from the studies discussed above to a large extent reflect the changing theories used to explain what happens when people, or audiences, are exposed to the mass media. Early studies of the media, for example, adopted what Trowler (1996) refers to as the 'hypodermic model', which uses the medical metaphor of the hypodermic syringe to describe the action of the media on an audience; in this model, the media acts as the syringe, which is used to 'inject' a message (the drug) into an audience (the patient), which in turn is affected by the injected message in much the same way as an injected drug would affect a patient. Studies informed by this model will seek correlations between the content of the media and the changes in attitudes and behaviours among their audiences. It is a flawed model for many reasons; for example, it fails to take account of:

- an audience member's pre-existing attitudes and belief systems, which may, to extend the medical metaphor, provide 'resistance' or 'immunity' to the 'injected' message
- the fact that audience members are not homogeneous and may belong to different 'subgroups', including those of gender, culture, sexual orientation and socio-economic background, all of which may influence the ways in which they respond to the message.

Nevertheless, this model is still to be found in the mass media, especially when they are reporting crimes where the perpetrator's criminal actions are supposed to have been inspired by the content of mass media, and especially images of sex and violence in cinemas and on the television.

Normative approach

A supposedly more sophisticated approach to understanding media influence is the so-called 'normative approach' (Trowler 1996). According to this model, the response of an audience to a media message or representation tends to conform to the values and belief systems that regulate social interaction. Nevertheless, they can be influenced by the stance taken by what Katz and Lazarsfeld (1955) initially referred to as 'opinion leaders', people with authority because their views are respected. In other words, according to this model, audience responses are not passive; they are the product of a two-step process that involves receipt of the message followed by its consideration in the light of past personal experience, comments by other audience members, and those of opinion leaders. A more recent extension of this idea is the multi-step flow model (Trowler 1996), which acknowledges that there are probably many more than two successive stages involved in the social interpretation of media messages.

There are, as one might expect, a number of problems with the normative approach. For example:

- it probably overestimates the extent to which people are influenced in their responses by their environment; a criticism of the approach supported by the fact that people can and do break social norms, change and redefine them
- it fails to take account of the fact that social norms are not always based on consensus; they may be formulated by a powerful élite in society and imposed on other members against their will.

Nevertheless, the model has been influential in studies of the media, and researchers adopting this position tend to study social-group responses to the media, seeking to identify opinion leaders and how media messages are interpreted through social interaction.

Uses and gratification model

An alternative model that recognizes the diversity that exists among the individuals that constitute a media audience is the 'uses and gratification' model. One of the early proponents of this model said that it asks the question not 'what does the media do to people?' but 'what do people do with the media?' (Katz 1955, cited in Trowler 1996). It acknowledges that the individuals who constitute an audience may be accessing the media for very different purposes: to obtain different types of pleasure or to satisfy very different needs. McQuail (2000) and Lull (1990) suggest that these uses and gratifications may range from the simple needs for diversion and escape, or the punctuation of time and activity, through to the far more complex dimensions of social affiliation and the confirmation of our own personal identity. Such an approach shifts research away from the effects of the media on an audience to an examination of the needs that audience members are meeting when they use the media. Not surprisingly, like the other approaches described above, it has been criticized on a number of levels, including:

- its failure to address the question *why* people have particular needs and *why* they use the media to satisfy them
- its assumption that the needs the media are used to satisfy are formed independently of the media, and
- its failure to recognize the cultural and social context of needs creation, and the role of the media as institutions as a part of that process.

Interpretive model

Yet another model, the 'interpretative' model, sees the products of the media as 'texts', in much the same way that a book or a newspaper article is a 'text'. Thus, members of an audience become 'readers' of 'media texts', interpreting, reinterpreting, or even ignoring, the messages that the media may convey. However, as members of society, media audiences inhabit a world of different discourses and message systems (Pecheux 1982), and their reading of, and reaction to, media texts is informed by the many other texts and discourses they are exposed to (Fiske 1988).

Interpreting media texts

Trowler (1996) suggests that the reading of a media text is a three-stage process; first, there is *selective exposure*, where audience members engage in a selection process before exposing themselves to the media, often selecting media texts that they feel will contain messages with which they agree. The second stage involves *selective perception*, a process whereby audience members tend to identify with media messages that match their own position, overlooking those that don't. The third and final stage involves the process of *selective retention*, a process whereby audience members tend to remember only the media messages with which they agree, or consider to be true or valid.

Buckingham (1993) goes so far as to suggest that there are different levels of 'media literacy', (low and high) that will affect how far an audience member is able to take the interpretation process (high media literacy facilitating greater understanding and critical engagement with a media text than low media literacy). However, Morley (1992) suggests that, although the potential audience interpretations of media messages may be many and varied, there is nevertheless a 'preferred reading' or dominant media message structured according to the cultural contexts in which it is generated (i.e. the culture of the media institution composing the message) and consumed (i.e. the cultural context of the audience reading it); for example, while a news item may be capable of multiple interpretations, one of them will be more likely to be selected by an audience than another because of the way it is presented and the general culture of those who are exposed to it.

Although identified separately in the literature as the *structured interpretation model* (Trowler 1996), it is really an extension of the *interpretation model* rather than a departure from it. It, therefore, shares many of the weaknesses of its progenitor, including a tendency to:

- underestimate the robustness of media messages
- ignore the fact that media messages tend to be repeated frequently and so fail to take account of the cumulative affect they may have
- see media text interpretation as an isolated rather than social activity
- assume that attitudes and views are largely determined by the social groups people belong to.

However, it does highlight the complexity of the mass-media-audience interaction phenomenon; one that mirrors the complexity of the relationship between attitudes and behaviour explored in another chapter of this book. It also draws attention to the dangers of both seeing an audience as an amorphous mass and attempting to understand audiences' responses to the media by dividing them according to age, socio-economic, gender, ethnic or other groupings.

Conclusion

However, this has not prevented 'that small number of enthusiasts' (Warnes 1995) who research and monitor media representations of older adults from making some interesting observations; as Warnes points out, old age itself is changing and no two cohorts of older adults are likely to display the same characteristics. Marked differences can be detected in the educational, occupational and marital histories of older adults and in their economic and material resources. For example, in the USA the over-50s now control over fifty per cent of disposable income, giving them significant market power (Trowler 1996). Perhaps even more significantly, recent demographic changes mean that older adults in the industrialized West (those aged 55 years and over) will very soon have vastly greater electoral power than younger people, which may well enable them to exercise increasing influence over policy development as politicians become more and more dependent on them for gaining and maintaining political office (Age Concern 1999).

To a large extent, the present state of play in media research reflects the theoretical developments in the social sciences commonly referred to as the post-structuralist and post-modernist positions; perspectives that recognize that not only will *different individuals* perceive and react to the same media messages or representations in different ways, but that the *same person* will perceive and react differently in different contexts. Such a position makes any generalizations about the impact of media representations, including those related to old age and the older adult, virtually impossible. Nevertheless, older adults, who tend to have far more positive attitudes to ageing than media representations would suggest (Victor 1987), are themselves turning to the media as a means of challenging the negative representations of older adults. In magazines such as *The Oldie* and *Retirement Choice*, older adults have found a means of articulating and drawing attention to the needs and concerns of older adults that they feel are neglected or ignored by the media generally. Adopting such a strategy clearly suggests that older adults believe in the power of the media to influence an audience, a belief it would be difficult to challenge given our present state of knowledge.

References:

Age Concern (1999) Debate of the age: The millennium papers: Values and Attitudes in an Ageing Society. London: Age Concern.

Biggs S (1993) Understanding Ageism. Milton Keynes: Open University Press

Buckingham D (ed) (1993) Reading Audiences: Young people and the media. Manchester: Manchester University Press.

Dail P W (1988) Prime-time portrayals of older adults in the context of family life. The Gerontologist 28 (5) 700–706

Featherstone M & Wernick A (eds) (1995) Images of Ageing. London: Routledge

Fiske J (1988) Television Culture. London: Methuen.

Harris D K (1990) Sociology of Ageing. London: Harper & Row.

Itzin C (1984) The double jeopardy of ageism and sexism. In: Bromely D B (ed) Gerontolgy: Social and Behavioural Perspectives. London: Croom Helm pp. 170–184.

Katz E (1955) Mass Communications Research and the Study of Popular Culture, Studies in Communication 2. In: Trowler P (1996) Investigating Mass Media 2nd edn. London: Harper Collins.

Katz E and Lazarsfeld P (1955) Personal Influence. NYFP.

Lambert J (1984) The Image of the Elderly on TV. Cambridge: University of the Third Age.

Lull J (1990) Inside Family Viewing: Ethnographic Research on Television's Audiences. London: Routledge.

McQuail D (2000) Mass Communication Theory. 4th edn. London: SAGE Publications Inc.

Moore S (1993) A certain ageism. The Guardian. 2 13 August, 11. In: Featherstone and Wernick (1995) p. 108.

Morley D (1992) Television Audiences and Cultural Studies. London: Routledge.

Moss Z (1970) It hurts to be alive and obsolete. The ageing woman. In: R Morgan (ed.) Sisterhood is Powerful. New York: Random House.

Palmore E (1971) Attitudes toward ageing as shown in humour. The Gerontologist. 11: 181–186

Palmore E (1986) Attitudes toward ageing as shown in humour: a review. In: Nahemow L, McCluskey-Fawcett K A and McGhee P E (eds) Humor and aging. Orlando, Flo: Academic.

Pecheux (1982) Language, semantics and ideology. London: Macmillan.

Rrbye B (1995) Old age in mass media: Images and attitudes. http://www.nig.nl/congres/3rdeuropeancongress 1995/abstract/030–1051.html

Sontag S (1978) The double standard of ageing. In: Carver V and Liddiard P(eds) An Ageing Population. London: Hodder and Stoughton.

Signorelli S (1989) Television and conceptions about sex roles. Sex Roles 21 (5/6) 341–360

Trowler P (1996) Investigating Mass Media. 2nd edn. London: Harper Collins.

Victor C R (1987) Old Age in Modern Society: A Textbook of Social Gerontology London: Chapman & Hall.

Warnes T (1995) Social constructions of old age: Components of the cultural dimension. Http://www.nig.nl/congres/3rdeuropeancongress 1995/abstract/013–1016.html

CHAPTER 14

Living well in old age

NICKY HAYES

Introduction

There are several possible perspectives that may be taken on what 'living well' actually means, depending on whether the perspective is that of an individual, an organization or society as a whole. In order to start with an individual perspective on living well in old age, stop reading for a moment and make a few notes of what 'living well in old age' means to you.

Looking over your list, perhaps you have a vision of independence, a happy home, good health and prosperity? Perhaps also the idea of time meaningfully spent on specific activities, such as church or voluntary work, enjoying children and grandchildren, holidays and entertainment? You probably have some other ideas; depending on numerous individual factors, such as personality, background, culture and gender, each person will draw up their list in a different way, and include different specific criteria for their future 'good life'.

Living well in old age means different things to different people, and each person's experience of old age will be unique. You are unlikely to have put losses such as ill health, bereavement or reduced income that may occur in later life on your list. It is only realistic to acknowledge that change or loss may occur, but it is still possible to live well despite this. Whether an individual assesses their life as satisfactory depends very much on how they adjust to and cope with the changes and losses that can occur. Some aspects of life can also be modified or influenced to varying extents; the next section will explore how it may be possible to promote health and prevent disability in later life.

Hughes (1993) has summarized the broad categories of elements that affect quality of life and these are reproduced in Box 14.1.

The number of elements identified in this list suggest that the concept of quality of life is a complex one. The implications arising from this list

212

Box 14.1: Factors contributing to quality of life

---

individual characteristics of old people
e.g. functional abilities, physical and mental health, dependency, personal characteristics such as gender, race and class

physical environmental factors
e.g. facilities and amenities, standards of housing, control over environment, comfort, security, regime in care settings

social environmental factors
e.g. levels of social and recreational activity, family and social networks, contact with organizations

socio-economic factors
e.g. income, nutrition, standard of living, socio-economic status

personal autonomy factors
e.g. ability to make choices, exercise control, negotiate environment

subjective satisfaction
the quality of life as assessed by the individual older person

personality factors
psychological well-being, morale, life satisfaction, affect, happiness

(from Hughes 1993)

---

extend beyond the experiences of individuals to policy and planning issues and associated legal and ethical considerations. The point is that quality of life is not just what the individual says it is; factors that may contribute to quality of life, such as standards of health, environment and nutrition are also both defined and influenced by society, services and policy makers. These definitions may be set higher or lower than where an individual might set them. For example, the standard and availability of hospital food was criticized by patients and relatives in the Health Advisory Service report (HAS 2000).

The concept is multi-layered and complex, and there is unlikely to be a panacea for old age, which guarantees that we shall all feel that we are living well. Much of this chapter will be concerned with discussing health issues, which can offer some pointers towards living well, but may not apply to every individual. Health and circumstances may be negotiable for some people, for other people they are not. For others, health is not a primary concern. For this reason the context of this chapter is living well, not just living healthily.

Living well – good health

Good health contributes to older people's quality of life and sense of living well. This section identifies and explores health issues relating to the prevention or reduction of the impact of chronic disease and disability, linking this to demographic issues, individual experience and policy issues.

Demographic issues relating to the health of older people

Analysis of future population trends informs policy and planning of health and social services for older people. The availability and quality of these services will in turn influence the circumstances and health of older people. Future population changes are predicted due to factors such as a falling birth rate, ageing of the cohort of people born in the early 1960s (the so-called 'baby boomers'), and increased life expectancy (Evandrou 1997).

Looking first at the ageing of the population as a whole, the expected trends may be summarized (Dargie 1999):

a. Between 1998 and 2015, the population of the United Kingdom is forecast to increase from 59 million people to 61.5 million. This is a relatively small rate of increase, which is likely to continue until 2025. After 2025, the population will start to decline.
b. After 2020, when the 'baby boomers' of the 1960s reach retirement age, there will be approximately 300 people of pension age per 1000 people. The number of retired people will rise to nearly 400 per 1000 by 2036, assuming that the state retirement age remains static.

Statistical analyses of future population trends do not, of course, reflect the diversity that exists within a population. With respect to the health of individuals, the proportion of older people in the population as a whole will not in itself cause increased health problems. It is the implications of population trends for policy and planning that may affect health, for example if insufficient services are planned to meet the specific health needs of older people.

The concept of life expectancy has more direct implications for the health of individual older people than the population statistics discussed above would suggest. This is because the longer a person lives, the more likely they are to develop a chronic or acute health problem, or a disability. Put another way, a person's *healthy* life expectancy is the number of years that they can expect to live without a chronic or disabling condition. This is not the same as a person's *total* life expectancy.

Table 14.1 shows the total-life expectancies and healthy-life expectancies of men and women in 1998. It can be seen that the average man might expect to have approximately fifty-nine years of *healthy* life and the average woman might expect to have approximately sixty-two years of *healthy* life.

Table 14.1: Life Expectancy

	Total life expectancy (years)	*Healthy life expectancy (years)*
Men	74.6	59
Women	79.7	62

Office of National Statistics (1998b)

It could be argued that averages such as these do not necessarily reflect individual experience. (We have all heard of, or know, someone who has lived to ninety or one hundred years and has rarely experienced ill health.) The average reflects the 'average' person, who may exist, but may not apply to us all individually. On the other hand, the average life expectancy of a population does affect us by the way in which the forecasts of the number of people surviving into later life are used. The forecasts of average life expectancy and healthy life expectancy affect policy and service provision and, in that way, are likely to filter back down to affect individuals.

Bearing in mind the disadvantages of discussing averages, the years of both healthy and unhealthy life are relevant to this discussion of living well. Healthy older people may be interested in how their health may be improved or maintained. Unhealthy years of life are of great importance to both the individual experiencing them and policy makers and service providers who aim to meet the health needs of these individuals and to 'add life to years'. The next section will identify some of the causes of unhealthy life years and will explore ways in which problems arising from them may be prevented or reduced.

Chronic disease and disability

As people reach old age, they are more likely to experience the onset of chronic disease than when they were younger. In fact, sixty-four per cent of men over the age of seventy-five, and sixty-eight per cent of women over the age of seventy-five report a long-standing illness, compared with twenty-seven per cent of men and women aged sixteen to forty-four (Office of National Statistics 1998a).

Chronic disease may result in a loss of function, such as reduced mobility, with a consequent reduction in the person's ability to independently manage daily living activities. In other words, chronic disease may result in years of unhealthy life and disability. The major causes of disability in old age are identified by Howse and Prophet (2000) as follows:

- arthritis or rheumatism
- osteoporosis
- cardiovascular disease
- respiratory disease
- dementia
- depression
- sensory impairment
- incontinence
- falls.

The causes of disability listed above include chronic diseases that arise from a range of causes throughout life, which may be beyond the control of the individual, such as environmental pollution. Because of this, it is not always possible for the disease to be reversed or cured in old age. This is why it is important to think about how the consequences of chronic disease, such as disability or chronic pain, might be relieved or reduced, as well as seeking to find treatments that will relieve or halt the chronic diseases themselves.

The above list identifies the main causes of disability in old age, although it does not illustrate the impact these have on how people manage daily activities, such as getting around, bathing and getting in and out of bed. Table 14.2 draws on statistical survey information to show the difficulty of accomplishing selected activities of people aged sixty-five and over in the United Kingdom. This gives a broad illustration of the type of impact that chronic health problems may have on older people.

The information in Table 14.2 indicates that despite the high level of reporting of long-standing illness the majority of older people manage these basic activities independently, although there is a significant minority of people who do not manage very well, many of whom are likely to be over the age of eighty-five. For people who have difficulty with activities of living, the consequences for their quality of life could be significant. For instance, should the person become housebound, there is less opportunity for social contact and a number of activities (Lindsay and Thompson 1993).

The list of major causes of disability, together with the information in Table 14.2, provides a sketch of potential health and functional problems in later life. An example of a more specific cause of difficulties is foot problems. Grundy et al (1997) found that foot problems are consistently associated with chronic difficulties experienced by older people. This may be due to chronic diseases, such as arthritis, rheumatism or diabetes, or general functional difficulty with toenail cutting. For example, it has been reported that sixty per cent of people over the age of eighty-five cannot cut their own toenails (Office of National Statistics

Table 14.2: Difficulty accomplishing selected activities of daily living (ADLs) in people aged sixty-five and over (percentage of people in each category)

Task	1994/1995 % of people in category
Difficulty managing stairs	
On own no difficulty	72
On own with some difficulty	19
Only with help or not at all	9
Difficulty going out of doors and walking down the road	
On own no difficulty	77
On own with some difficulty	10
Only with help or not at all	13
Difficulty bathing	
On own no difficulty	82
On own with some difficulty	10
Only with help or not at all	8
Difficulty getting around the house	
On own no difficulty	91
On own with some difficulty	8
Only with help or not at all	1
Difficulty getting in or out of bed	
On own no difficulty	92
On own with some difficulty	6
Only with help or not at all	2

from: Jarvis (1997)

1996). This might suggest that there is a case for toenail cutting and chiropody services for older people to be more widely available or accessible. This is, of course, partly a policy issue and will be returned to later in the discussion.

Reducing disability due to chronic health problems

It was noted above that it is important to proceed beyond the identification of causes and types of disability to the identification of how disability may be prevented or reduced. Returning to the list of causes of disability that were identified earlier, some evidence for the prevention of chronic disease or reduction of disability in older people is summarized below.

Arthritis and rheumatism

Arthritis is a very common form of disability amongst people over the age of sixty-five. There is no specific curative treatment available, and treatment is therefore aimed at symptomatic relief. Arthritis is a complex disease that can affect the whole person, due to pain, restriction in activity and distress. Holman and Lorig (1997) stress the importance of coping mechanisms, including the proper use of medication and exercise to improve symptoms and limit progression. Fries (1992) suggests that a reduction of obesity through diet and exercise may prevent or relieve the condition.

Osteoporosis

Osteoporosis may affect both men and women, although it is more common in women partly because of bone loss due to the menopause. Risk factors include smoking, physical inactivity and high alcohol consumption. A 'silent epidemic', osteoporosis is a hidden problem that may not be noticed until fractures and consequent disability occur. Prevention of osteoporosis is an important issue for health promotion earlier in life and middle age. Chapuy et al (1992) suggest that bone loss and risk of fracture in older women may be reduced by calcium supplements. Diet should be the first source of calcium. The National Osteoporosis Society (2000) recommend a calcium intake for women over the age of forty-five (not taking hormone replacement therapy) and men over the age of sixty-five of 1500 mg per day. This is equivalent to consuming just over two pints of milk per day. Curl (2000) recommends that women maintain an active lifestyle as they age to maintain bone mineral density and prevent osteoporosis.

Cardiovascular disease

Coronary heart disease is the leading cause of death in the United Kingdom. After heart disease and cancer, strokes are the third most common cause. It is now well established that prevention strategies aimed at smoking cessation, reducing obesity, high blood pressure, serum glucose and cholesterol and increasing activity may reduce the risk of these diseases. It is well worth people continuing to address these risk factors in old age as well as earlier in life. For example, reducing salt and saturated fat intake is effective in lowering blood pressure in older people and may greatly affect cardiovascular disease (Law et al 1991a, Law et al 1991b). The medical treatment of existing high blood pressure is also effective in reducing heart disease and the risk of strokes in older people (Sanderson 1996, Mulrow et al 1997). Standard health advice currently encourages people of all ages to consume five portions of fruit and vegetables per day, and it has been found that increasing fruit and vegetables by one to two servings per day may protect against strokes in men (Gillman et al 1995).

Respiratory disease

There is evidence to suggest that stopping smoking even well into middle age results in a reduction in the subsequent risk of lung cancer (Peto et al 2000). Older smokers may have smoked for many years, and may find it difficult to quit, but there are health benefits to be gained from doing so. Raw et al (1998) suggest that support and encouragement of nicotine-replacement therapy are effective methods to help people stop smoking. Respiratory disease in older people may also be reduced by use of the influenza vaccine (Gross et al 1995).

Sensory impairment

It is thought that official estimates of the number of older people with visual or hearing impairment underestimate the number of people who experience difficulties (Bruce et al 1991, Wilson et al 1993). It may be suggested that there are numerous reasons why older people do not report problems or seek treatment: they may find their own ways of coping, they may have low expectations ('it's just my age'), there may be a lack of information about services or access may be difficult, or they may have a low opinion of the services on offer.

Sensory impairment may lead to disability, particularly outside the home, because shops or public buildings are often not user-friendly to older people who have visual or hearing impairments.

Visual impairment

The most common causes of visual impairment in old age are macular degeneration, cataracts, glaucoma and diabetic retinopathy. Cataracts cannot be prevented or retarded by any currently known medical or dietary measures, although it has been suggested that the use of UVB blocking sunglasses in bright sunlight may influence cataract development (Kalina 1997). Screening and treatments are available for other problems such as glaucoma and diabetic retinopathy.

Overall, it can be suggested that early detection and treatment are extremely important for problems such as glaucoma, cataracts, macular degeneration and diabetic retinopathy in order to prevent or reduce disability due to visual impairment. When people develop non-correctable visual impairment, the development of coping strategies and appropriate use of assistive equipment are important. Advice and help is also available in the UK from voluntary organisations or charities, such as the Royal National Institute for the Blind and the Partially Sighted Society.

Hearing impairment

Hearing loss is often a 'hidden disability', because the person looks 'normal' and may not draw attention to their impairment. It can be disabling and adversely affect their quality of life in many ways, such as making communication difficult or promoting a lack of confidence, social isolation, and bringing about a reduced enjoyment of leisure activities, such as listening to music or television. The age-related type of hearing loss is not currently specifically preventable, although Gate and Rees (1997) suggest that maintaining good general health will minimize the loss of hearing due to systemic disease, such as hypertension, hyperlipidaemia and diabetes. Hearing impairment is most frequently treated by giving the patient a hearing aid, although problems with hearing aids are common (Wilson et al 1993), such as distortion.

Incontinence

Incontinence is not an inevitable consequence of the ageing process. Urinary incontinence can be treated, for example there is evidence to suggest that urinary-urge incontinence may be treated by bladder training, although further, larger trials are needed on this (Roe et al 1999). More research evidence is also needed on prevention strategies. Fonda et al (1999 p. 760) suggest that prevention strategies fall into three categories, with secondary prevention more likely to be achievable than primary prevention:

- primary prevention – prevents predisposing condition (e.g. childbirth trauma)
- secondary prevention – reverses predisposing condition or prevents progression of condition into incontinence
- tertiary prevention – management strategies to decrease the severity or sequelae of incontinence, such as skin irritation and social restriction.

Falls

The main risk factors for falls in older people are loss of muscle strength and flexibility, and impaired balance and reaction time (Myers et al 1996). These may be due to neurological disorders, dementia, undesired effects of some medication, alcohol consumption, physical illness, physical disability or hazards within or outside the home. It is desirable to reduce the risk of falls. This will reduce their unwanted consequence: the pain and distress experienced by older people who have sustained fractures, and the considerable financial cost to the NHS. For example, there are 60,000 hip fractures in England and Wales each year occupying 25% of all orthopaedic beds (Armstrong and Wallace 1994). Given the increase in the age-specific rate of hip fracture and the predicted increase in the older population, there could be as many as 96,000 new hip fractures in England and Wales by the year 2031, requiring an additional 1.6 million extra bed-days and £507 million in direct hospital costs alone (Hollingworth et al 1995). There is now plenty of evidence to suggest that exercise programmes for older people to improve factors, such as strength and balance, can be effective in prevention (Tinetti 1994, Campbell et al 1997). As with many other factors related to healthy living, maintaining activity levels is important for all older people, whether as part of a planned exercise programme or through regular daily exercise such as walking. Preventing environmental hazards is also important, particularly within the home, to try to avoid problems that may be compounded by sensory impairment.

Stairs are particularly hazardous to the old, and care should be taken that stairways used by older people are well lit, have clearly visible step edges and do not have repetitive carpet patterns that may produce a false perception in those with defective visual fixation. Stairways can also be hazardous if there are irregularities in the height or depth of treads or any other features that require a change in the natural rhythm of walking (World Health Organisation 1989 p. 39).

The above discussion has presented a selection of the evidence for the prevention of disability and the promotion of healthy living in old age. Drawing on this evidence, a simple package of health advice, which is relevant to all older people, is summarized in Table 14.3.

Policy issues

The toenail-cutting example (see p. 217) raises general issues about services and information for older people who are seeking to live well. There are two fundamental issues involved: one is that of resources for services and the other is that of the right of older people to choose whether they accept these services or not.

On the first issue, it is clear that, with a forecasted increase in the proportion of older people in the population of the UK, policy issues

Table 14.3: Health advice for older people

Preventative action	Potential effects
Diet	
Consumption of five or more servings of fruit and vegetables per day	Preventative role against problems including cardiovascular disease, cancers, diverticular disease, presbyacusis and diabetes
Consumption of 1500 mg calcium daily (equivalent to approximately two pints of milk)	Prevent osteoporosis
Reduce obesity	Relieve symptoms of osteoarthritis
Smoking cessation	Reduces risk of problems such as lung cancer, cardiovascular disease, respiratory disease, osteoporosis, macular degeneration
Reduce salt intake	Reduce risk of cardiovascular disease
Increase physical activity (minimum of twenty minutes exercise, such as walking three times a week)	Preventive role against falls, cardiovascular disease, osteoporosis Relieves symptoms of osteoarthritis
Moderate alcohol consumption	Reduces risk of falls, accidents and osteoporosis

related to financing healthcare will remain important in the twenty-first century. In the 1990s awareness of the potential costs of healthcare for older people encouraged a policy focus on living well *into* old age, that is the prevention of ill health in later life through interventions aimed at younger people. For example, the White Paper 'Saving Lives: Our Healthier Nation' (DOH 1999) focuses strategies on, and targets for, the under seventy-fives.

The needs of older people were more directly addressed in subsequent policy documents (DOH 2000, Audit Commission 2000), which identified the need and resources for rehabilitation and intermediate care services (see Note 1 p. 228). Rehabilitation involves the restoration (to the maximum degree possible) either of the function (physical or mental) or the role (within the family, social network or workforce) of the older person (Nocon and Baldwin 1998). When rehabilitation is effective, it helps an individual to live well, because they have recovered from an illness, disability has been prevented, or they have learnt to cope with an impairment. From a service perspective, there is also an incentive in reducing costly hospital stays and the problem of 'bed blocking'; in other words, there is a resource incentive for developing these services.

'Effective rehabilitation can help people to stay at home, or return home after hospital and reduce admissions to residential and nursing homes. It requires a range of services' (Audit Commission 2000 p. 1).

Dargie's (1999) analysis of the future for healthcare policy in the UK supports the view that there is likely to be a continuing policy emphasis on encouraging lifestyle changes, such as stopping smoking, having a healthy diet and adequate exercise. She further points out that the picture is complicated by the health inequalities that underlie national data: there is a need to tackle associated problems, such as unemployment, deprivation and poor education, which affect the health and well-being of people in all age groups in the population. The concept of living well is a complex one. Health and social policy is frequently fluid, and the extent to which these factors are addressed may depend upon politics, public opinion and electoral issues, which are not necessarily directly related to rigorous research findings.

The second issue raised was that of the individual's right to choose whether they wish to improve their health and, if so, whether they wish to use services that are available. The concept of empowerment is closely related to this issue. It could be suggested that, in an ideal situation, health-related choices are made in the way described by Hopson and Scally (cited Brown and Parker 1995 p. 118):

> Self-empowerment means ... having the abilities to identify the alternatives in any
> situation, [and] to choose one on the basis of one's values, priorities, and commit-
> ments. None of the alternatives in some situations may be desirable, but it is the
> knowledge that there is always a choice that heralds the beginning of self-empowered
> thinking.

These choices would include whether to seek medical or other health services or whether to follow health advice. The issues relating to choice and empowerment are complex, owing to the diversity of health beliefs of older age groups and the way that decision-making is shaped. Ford (1986) suggests that the decision to seek medical aid 'is shaped by culture, attitudes, folk medical knowledge, personal biography, influence from social networks, present goals and perceptions of the costs and benefits of entering the "sick role" as well as by the inherent ambiguity of most symptoms themselves'.

According to this view, people may be aware of services or assistance that is being offered, but it may not meet their need or expectation. This suggestion is supported by evidence that non-specific, general health-education services or campaigns aimed at changing behaviours do not significantly reduce disease and mortality (Ebrahim and Davey-Smith 1997). The exception to this seems to be counselling people who are at risk of coronary heart disease, a specific health intervention that has been found to be effective (Steptoe et al 1999). In general terms, it can be suggested that older people as a group are more receptive to recommendations for healthy living than younger people, particularly for diet, blood pressure monitoring and home safety (Heidrich 1998). This strengthens the argument for organizations to offer health advice to older people, particularly to 'at risk' groups; whether people follow this advice is then a matter of individual choice.

The issues relating to choice and empowerment reflect the complexity of living well in old age. The next section will address some of the social and environmental issues related to living well.

Good living – good health in context

At the beginning of this chapter, it was demonstrated that living well means more than just maintaining good physical health. Hughes' list of the elements that make up quality of life included social and environmental factors as well as many individual factors and characteristics, of which health was just one. The list you may have made of your criteria for living well probably included a number of these elements too. This section will briefly consider some of these other factors, focusing on individual coping strategies, and social and environmental factors.

Individual coping strategies

It was suggested earlier that if change or losses occur in later life, individual factors shape people's reactions to events and influence how they cope. From an individual developmental perspective, Erikson's theory (see Chapter 7) suggests that the way in which people adjust to old age partly depends upon past experiences and conflicts and how these have been resolved earlier in life. From this it might be inferred that if an older person has not felt in control of situations or changes earlier in life, or has not satisfactorily dealt with subsequent feelings of impotence, they may lack coping strategies in some situations later on. It could be suggested that adverse social or environmental factors compound feelings of helplessness, lack of choice and lack of control. For an example of a social factor, Grant (1996) suggests that ageism can often affect the choices people are presented with and the decisions they make about those choices. The relationship of environmental factors to coping strategies is discussed below.

Environment – institution or home

Most older people live independently in their own home. The saying 'home is where the heart is' may be a cliché, but it also sums up the subjective meaning of having somewhere to identify with, be comfortable, be sociable, and invest with meanings and feelings. Draper (1997) identifies home as a locus for autonomy, a place where choice is maximally available. For many people, remaining independent in their own home remains their preferred choice of where to spend old age, and enhances their quality of life. But, as Harding (1997) points out, housing must be warm, safe and convenient. With the minimum income for people claiming the state pension at £75 per week for a single person (at the time of writing), it can be difficult for older owner-occupiers to maintain a good standard of repair and comfort. Harding argues for the development of a strategy for housing improvement. This includes addressing financial assistance, and re-examining the scope of older people's involvement in the planning process. This relates back to the type of policy and demographic issues raised in the previous section on policy issues.

For a minority of people, one of the major changes that they might face in old age is a move from their own home into residential care. For older people in hospital or living in residential care, the physical environment they are in may no longer be embedded with the meanings they associate with 'home', and there may well no longer be the same kind of freedom that they have at home.

Researcher: But what do you like about being at home though?

Mrs C: Being able to please yourself. Freedom of being able to choose what you do and what you eat. You see, you can't do that in hospital. (Draper 1997 p. 107)

A move to residential care may be a positive experience for people, improving their quality of life due to social, comfort and safety factors, and assisted by the coping mechanisms of the individual. For others, the process may not be so positive, resulting in a stress that might even prove fatal (Coffman 1981). It could be argued that this is a particularly difficult life change to make if the move is preceded by a stay in hospital due to a health crisis. At such a time as this the person may be feeling vulnerable and not very well equipped to make major decisions. It is of paramount importance that the individuals concerned are involved as much as possible in these decisions and provided with information and choice. The consequences of moves into nursing homes or other institutional care may then be less traumatic and even result in lower mortality rates after the move (Gutman and Herbert 1976).

When moving into residential care, a person's familiar home is lost, probably along with personal possessions, all of which have important meanings for them. The extent to which individuals feel loss in this type of situation may be considerable, as illustrated by the poem in Box 14.2.

While it is impossible to generalize about how and where people wish to live as they get older, there is no doubt that meanings and feelings are individual and important, even though they may not be expressed as clearly and articulately as they are in Mrs Barnes' poem. It is particularly important for workers in institutional care settings to be aware of what factors may contribute to quality of life, and to acknowledge the adjustments that people may have to make when they move into residential care. This may sound obvious, but, as Oleson et al (1994) found in their study of nursing homes in southwest England, nurses and residents may differ in their perceptions of what things are important to the residents' quality of life, and what nursing interventions help to promote a good quality of life.

Relationships

Old age, change or loss does not automatically make people unhappy or lonely. Some people may be happy despite chronic health problems or the loss of their home. It is often other people that make the difference – one important factor in living well is the relationships that people have with family and friends. Grundy et al's (1997) study of what sustains well-being and quality of life found that between sixty-eight and seventy-three per cent of people over the age of sixty-five were happy with their overall

Box 14.2: *The Day Room* by Wyn Barnes

Is this our hell?
In clean white buildings, in our padded chairs,
With cups of tepid tea and telly blaring
And people silent, slumped like dolls
Each wrapped in the impenetrable web
Of his own misery.

Is this our hell?
The grief
For loss of home and family and pets:
Our inability to choose
To walk, to sit: the simplest act
Beyond out failing powers.

Is this our hell?
This crowded solitude;
We are too old, too deaf, too locked in pain
To comfort one another.
Strangers we were at first,
Strangers remain.

Is this our hell?
Bland nurses come and go
With 'Darling', 'Love', and strong, impatient arms.
Their god-like power
Can notice or ignore our call
And grumble when we cannot wait.

Their world extends
To home and children, washing, gardens, sex
And cuddles, cats and cars.
Were we once like them?

Now, hauled like sacks, toileted, Christian-named,
Our useless limbs
Full of unheeded aches,
We wait and sleep and eat
In desolate comfort, lonely crowded rooms.

Not to be known
As once we were
Wife, mother, worker, friend,
But only as this useless hulk
That is our hell.

included with kind permission of Wyn Barnes

quality of life, and that most people were well supported by family and friends. People aged eighty-five and over with poor life satisfaction were those most likely to have the fewest relatives, friends and confidants. The relationships with family and friends are tremendously important to many people throughout life; therefore, it is not surprising that they remain so in old age. People who have confiding relationships cope better with change and loss in old age, that is they are less vulnerable to negative events in later life (Murphy 1982).

For people living alone, as well as direct human contact, company can come in many guises, such as a loved pet, the radio or television. The increasing availability and use of computers and the Internet is also likely to offer opportunities for contact and communication for older people who are not able to get out as much as they used to.

This section has only very briefly looked at some important factors that form the context of living well. It may be suggested that health and social care workers need to be aware of the changes and range of losses that people may face in old age and of the part that both the individual and others may play in shaping these experiences into ones that may be lived well. There are many grounds for a positive outlook on old age – it is not all doom and gloom, and most people do live happily and independently into old age.

Conclusions

This chapter has identified a number of factors that relate to the concept of 'living well' in old age. The key factors of health, environment, relationships and individual differences and coping mechanisms have been identified, with a focus on how good health and the prevention of chronic disease and disability may be approached. The discussion has focused on physical health, but mental health is also vital for living well – this has been discussed in depth in Chapter 8. The evidence suggests that, by eating a good diet, maintaining activity and stopping smoking, older people may continue to maximize their chances of good health and reduce the risk of disability due to chronic health problems such as heart disease, strokes, cancer, musculo-skeletal diseases, sensory impairment, incontinence and falls.

There is more to good living than just health. Because of this, people's different personalities and outlooks on life have been implicit throughout this discussion of living well: the background, culture and gender differences that shape people and the opportunities they face and the choices they make. How people cope with change and the losses that may occur in later life are emergent factors of the complexity of living well in old age.

The environment that people live in, the meaning that they attach to their home, and the relationships they maintain have also been seen to be important elements of a good quality of life.

The context of health and social policy issues has also been explored. These issues affect people's lives, both directly and indirectly, owing to the increasing likelihood of chronic health problems in later life. It has been shown that UK policy trends are now beginning to align with the maintenance of health and independence in old age, including a trend towards further development of rehabilitation and intermediate services for older people.

It can be concluded that, while each individual may take responsibility and use opportunities for living as well as possible in later life, there are many personal, social and environmental factors that contribute to living well, which may or may not be amenable to control by the individual. Health and social policy also has a role to play in ensuring that the needs of older people are addressed and met. If older people need to use services, it is important that health and social care workers understand the uniqueness of each person and what living well means to them.

Note

[1] Intermediate services are described by the Audit Commission (2000) as meeting 'a range of needs for the medically stable with a focus on "confidence building". Can be used post-discharge (step-down) or as a half-way house between home and hospital (step-up)'.

References

Armstrong A L, Wallace W A (1994) The epidemiology of hip fractures and methods of prevention. Acta Orthop Belg; 60 Suppl 1: 85–101.

Audit Commission (2000) The Way to Go Home: rehabilitation and remedial services for older people. London: Audit Commission.

Brown P A and Parker S M (1995) Empowerment or social control? Differing interpretations of psychology in health education. Health Education Journal 54 (1): 115–123.

Bruce I, McKennell A and Walker E (1991) Blind and partially sighted adults in Britain: the RNIB survey. London: HMSO.

Campbell A J, Robertson M C, Gardner M M, Norton R N, Tilyard M W and Buchner D M (1997) Randomised controlled trial of a general practice programme of home based exercise to prevent falls in elderly women. British Medical Journal 315 (7115): 1065–1069.

Chapuy M C, Arlot M E Duboeuf F, Brun J, Crouzet B, Arnaud S, Delmas P D and Meunier P J (1992) Vitamin D3 and calcium to prevent hip fractures in elderly women. New England Journal of Medicine 327 (23): 1637–1642.

Coffman T (1981) Relocation and survival of institutionalised aged: a re-examination of the evidence. Gerontologist 21 (5): 483–500.

Curl W W (2000) Ageing and exercise: are they compatible in women? Clinical Orthopaedics and Related Research 372: 151–158.

Dargie C (1999) Policy Futures for UK Health No. 3 Demography: analysing trends and policy issues in births, deaths and diseases for the UK population in 2015. London: Nuffield Foundation.

DOH (1999) Saving Lives: Our Healthier Nation. London: HMSO.

DOH (2000) The NHS Plan: A plan for investment, A plan for reform. London: HMSO.

Draper P (1997) Nursing Perspectives on Quality of Life. London: Routledge.

Ebrahim S and Davey Smith G (1997) Systematic review of randomised controlled trials of multiple risk factor interventions for preventing coronary heart disease. British Medical Journal 314 (7095): 1666–1674.

Evandrou M (1997) Baby Boomers: Ageing in the Twenty-first Century. London: Age Concern.

Fonda D, Benvenuti F, Castleden M, Cottenden A et al (1999) Management of Incontinence in Older People. In: Abrams P, Khoury S, Wein A (eds) Incontinence. First International Consultation on Incontinence pp. 735–760. Plymouth: Health Publication Ltd.

Ford G G (1986) Illness behaviour in the elderly. In: Dean K, Hickey T and Holstein B E (eds) Self-care and Health in Old Age. Health Behaviour. Implications for Policy and Practice pp. 130–166. London: Croom Helm.

Fries J (1992) Strategies for the reduction of morbidity. American Journal of Clinical Nutrition 55: 1257S–1262S.

Gate G A and Rees T S (1997) Successful Auditory Aging. Western Journal of Medicine 167 (4): 247–252.

Gillman M W, Cupples L A, Gagnon D, Posner B M, Ellison R C, Castelli W P and Wolf P A (1995) Protective effect of fruits and vegetables on development of stroke in men. Journal of the American Medical Association 273 (14): 1113–1117.

Grant L D (1996) Effects of ageism on individual and healthcare providers' responses to healthy ageing. Health and Social Work 21 (1): 9–15.

Gross P A, Hermogenes A W and Sacks H S (1995) The efficacy of influenza vaccine in elderly persons. A meta-analysis and review of the literature. Annals of Internal Medicine 123 (7): 518–27.

Grundy E, Bowling A and Farqhar M (1997) Living Well into Old Age. London: Age Concern/Joseph Rowntree Foundation.

Gutman G and Herbert C (1976) Mortality rates among extended-care patients. Journal of Gerontology 31: 352–357.

Harding T (1997) A Life Worth Living: the independence and inclusion of older people. London: Help the Aged.

HAS (2000) Not because they are old – an independent inquiry into the care of older people on acute wards in general hospitals. London: Health Advisory Service.

Heidrich S M (1998) Health promotion in old age. Annual Review of Nursing Research 16: 173–195.

Hollingworth W, Todd CJ Parker MJ (1995) The cost of treating hip fractures in the twenty-first century. J Public Health Med; 17: 269–276.

Holman H R and Lorig K R (1997) Overcoming Barriers to Successful Aging, self-management of osteoarthritis. Western Journal of Medicine 167 (4): 265–268.

Howse K and Prophet H (2000) Improving the Health of Older Londoners: reviewing the evidence. London: Centre for Policy on Ageing.

Hughes B (1993) Gerontological approaches to quality of life. In: Johnson J and Slater R (eds) Ageing in Later Life. London: Sage Publications.

Jarvis C (1997) Past, present and future trends in old age morbidity in Great Britain. Working Paper Number 10. London: Age Concern Institute of Gerontology.

Kalina R E (1997) Seeing into the future – vision and ageing. Western Journal of Medicine 167 (4): 253–257.

Law M R, Frost C D and Wald N J (1991a) By how much does dietary salt reduction lower blood pressure? I – Analysis of observational data among populations. British Medical Journal 302 (6780): 811–815.

Law M R, Frost C D and Wald N J (1991b) By how much does dietary salt reduction lower blood pressure? III – Analysis of data from trials of salt reduction. British Medical Journal 302 (6780): 819–824.

Lindsay J and Thompson C (1993) Housebound elderly people: definition, prevalence and characteristics. International Journal of Geriatric Psychiatry 8: 231–237.

Mulrow C, Lau J, Cornell J, Brand M and Amato M (1997) Antihypertensive therapy in the elderly (Cochrane Review). The Cochrane Library Oxford, Update Software.

Murphy E (1982) Social origins of depression in old age. British Journal of Psychiatry 141: 135–142.

Myers A H, Young Y and Langlois J A (1996) Prevention of falls in the elderly. Bone 18 (1 supplement 1): 87S–101S.

National Osteoporosis Society http://www.nos.org.uk/prevent.htm

Nocon A and Baldwin S (1998) Trends in Rehabilitation Policy – a Literature Review. London: Kings Fund.

Office of National Statistics (1996) Living in Britain: results from the 1994 General Household Survey. London: HMSO.

Office of National Statistics (1998a) Living in Britain: results from the 1996 General Household Survey. London: HMSO.

Office of National Statistics (1998b) Social Trends 28. London: HMSO.

Oleson M, Heading C, McGlynn K and Bistodeau J A (1994) Quality of life in long-stay institutions in England: nurse and resident perceptions. Journal of Advanced Nursing 20 (1): 23–32.

Peto R, Darby S, Deo H, Silcocks P, Whitley E and Doll R (2000) Smoking, smoking cessation, and lung cancer in the UK since 1950: combination of national statistics with two case-control studies. British Medical Journal 321 (7257): 323–329.

Raw M, McNeill A and West R (1998) Smoking cessation guidelines for health professionals. A guide to effective smoking cessation interventions for the healthcare system. Thorax 53 (supplement 5) 1, S1–19.

Roe B, Williams K and Palmer M (1999) Training for urinary incontinence in adults (Cochrane Review) In: The Cochrane Library, issue 3, 2000, Oxford: Update Software

Sanderson S (1996) Hypertension in the elderly: pressure to treat? Health Trends 28 (4): 117–121.

Steptoe A, Doherty S, Rink E, Kerry S, Kendrick T and Hilton S. (1999) Behavioural Counselling in general practice for the promotion of healthy behaviour among adults at increased risk of coronary heart disease: randomised trial. British Medical Journal 319 (7215): 943–947.

Tinetti M E, Baker D I, McAvay G, Claus E, Garrett P, Gottschalk M, Koch M L. Trainor K and Horwitz R I (1994) A multifactorial intervention to reduce the risk of falling among elderly people living in the community. New England Journal of Medicine 331 (13): 821–827.

Wilson P S, Fleming D M and Donaldson I (1993) Prevalence of hearing loss among people aged 65 years and over: screening and hearing aid provision. British Journal of General Practice 43 (375): 406–409.

World Health Organisation (1989) Health of the Elderly. Technical Report Series 779. Geneva: World Health Organisation.

Conclusion

Philip Woodrow

Introduction

Ageing is an inevitable part of the life span. Ageing begins with birth (or, arguably, conception) and continues until death. However, the main effects of ageing are likely to be more evident in the later years of life. Over the past two centuries, improvements in social conditions and medical progress have significantly reduced premature mortality. Together with a decline in birth rates, this has resulted in an 'ageing' society. The ageing of society may be especially evident in Western countries such as the UK but is occurring worldwide. An ageing society raises issues for:

- the individual
- healthcare
- society (as a whole).

This book has explored these issues from perspectives of biological, psychological and social ageing. This final chapter synthesizes these themes, identifying key issues for health and healthcare.

A common stereotype of ageing suggests disease, decline in function and dementia. Yet such stereotypes are usually applied to other people, seldom to ourselves. This was illustrated by the example given in Chapter 9 where one lady stated that she was in a ward because she was ill, while the others were there because 'they were old'. Age, and health, therefore, become relative concepts. Ageing includes the potential for disease, decline in function and dementia, but all of these could be considered *unhealthy ageing*, a negative approach to ageing. While healthcare should, as far as possible, provide whatever help is needed, a more positive approach to ageing is to promote *healthy ageing*. Healthy ageing is fundamentally about preventing as many problems as possible, and maximizing alternative functions where problems do occur. Healthy ageing, therefore, seeks to support the individual in their own environment, or as near-normal an environment as possible.

The individual

Stating that each person is an individual is stating the obvious. This obvious statement is included in almost any philosophy about health – almost everyone values their own individuality. Healthy ageing should therefore promote the individuality of each person. But health is a value-laden concept, and what one person considers 'healthy', another may not. Most old people consider themselves to be healthy (Tinker 1997).

Healthcare

Although almost all healthcare philosophies emphasize the importance of individuality, healthcare is provided through systems and institutions that attempt to provide equitable standards to everyone. While this is intended to promote fairness and equity, as identified in Chapter 10, healthcare structures tend to encourage conformity. Healthcare workers may, therefore, be caught in a conflict between individuality and conformity. Healthcare aims to promote healthy ageing; this aim is more likely to be achieved by encouraging healthcare institutions to recognize and overcome the constraints within which they work.

Society

Another obvious statement is that individuals and healthcare do not exist in a vacuum, but within a particular society and social structure. Individuals' views and expectations, and provision of healthcare, are influenced by the society within which they live. For example, healthcare policies and funding are strongly influenced by governmental priorities, which in turn are partly influenced by the desire of that government to remain in power. The values of a particular society will therefore influence governmental policy and funding. But the values of a society also influence individuals, which includes both healthcare recipients and healthcare providers/professionals. Understanding social values, therefore, provides a necessary context for understanding the dynamics that influence healthcare provision and expectations.

Measuring ageing

Chapter 1 outlines the framework for this book and establishes some of the main themes developed in subsequent chapters. Various perspectives to measure ageing are identified. Chronology, measuring age by the number of years lived, is widely used throughout society. Chronological age provides clear parameters for statistical analysis and so is frequently used for healthcare research and government data. For example, fairness in deciding eligibility for a state pension is achieved by it being related to chronological age. However, the number of years lived provides a poor measurement of someone's health status. In addition, using chronological age in this way can result in 'ageism' and other ethical problems. For example, healthcare resources designated specifically for older people, often with a minimum-age limit for access, can leave much to be desired. The value of chronological perspectives for this book is therefore rejected in Chapter 1, which identifies three key perspectives:

- physiological
- psychological
- sociological.

Each perspective forms a section of this book.

Physiological ageing

Physiological ageing measures age by someone's physiological function. The maximum function of almost all physiological systems declines with age. Physiological perspectives can therefore appear negative. However, in health each system at birth is able to function considerably beyond the minimum level needed to maintain homeostasis. This functional reserve will usually be sufficient to maintain adequate function for homeostasis of most systems throughout a human lifetime. So, although age-related changes occur to the body, (chronic) ill health is not a normal or inevitable result of the ageing process.

Chapter 2 explores the main, current theories of physiological ageing, including:

- Hayflick's 'biological clock'
- subsequent research surrounding apoptosis.

Understanding ageing can help promote healthy ageing, and enable health professionals to provide better care. Healthy ageing includes physical, as well as psychological and social, health. While problems can usually be better understood through reductionist approaches, such as exploring individual body systems, it is the whole person who is (or is not) healthy. Health can exist despite medical labels; so people with chronic diseases or limitations to physical abilities may consider themselves to be healthy. Theories attempting to explain the process of ageing may suggest ways in which individuals can age more healthily, but theories inevitably remain at best tentative and generalized. Modern science has sought to understand ageing so that it can achieve greater health, which includes providing better healthcare. So, although the physical body is only a part of the whole person/individual, achieving the best possible physical health is an important part of healthy ageing. Physiologically, healthy ageing can therefore be achieved despite chronic diseases or limitations to physical abilities.

Chapters 3–5 adopt a largely systems-based (reductionist) approach. Chapter 3 discusses bones, muscles and skin; Chapter 4 discusses the cardiovascular system; Chapter 5 provides a brief overview of other body systems. This reductionist approach provides a useful way to focus in some depth on the function of each system, how it is affected by ageing, causes of disease and possible treatments/management. Readers should use this knowledge in the context of both the individual and the whole person. So, someone does not simply have 'heart disease'; cardiac failure can affect other systems in the body, but may also affect their psychological and social health.

While ageing is not a disease, various disease processes do increasingly occur with age, including many chronic conditions that impair quality of life. Pathophysiology and possible therapeutic drugs and chemicals have been increasingly studied during recent years. For example, Chapter 3 identifies that:

- inadequate antioxidants
- inadequate apoptosis
- cytokines

have all been found in people with arthritis. Therefore, targeting these factors with drugs, such as interferon beta, could potentially alleviate, and possibly reverse, the pathological process. Currently, a range of novel drugs and therapies for various diseases is being tested. The past history of pharmacology suggests there are likely to be some false hopes and starts, but that some beneficial drugs will probably be identified for many problematic chronic conditions.

It is unrealistic to expect to remain free from illness throughout one's life. Diseases and illnesses can, and will almost inevitably, occur. Physiological illness is a result of some systems being unable to maintain the minimum function needed to maintain homeostasis. Disease may be acute or chronic. Some of the chronic diseases that more often occur among older people have been discussed in this book. However, this is not a book on pathophysiology; so health professionals are likely to encounter a range of other illnesses and problems that have not been identified here.

While function of one or more systems may decline, 'health' and 'disease' are concepts that can vary between individuals. Despite disease labels, people may consider themselves to be healthy. This is particularly important to remember with chronic problems. So, as people adjust to their limitations, they may accept that they have problems, but still consider themselves healthy. The danger of giving medical labels to problems is that unrealistic expectations, or pejorative stigmas, may be attached to them. Old age is not a disease, it cannot be cured, and it is ethically questionable whether anyone should wish to attempt to cure it. Age-related problems may be curable; if incurable, alleviation may be possible, such as pain relief. But healthcare also has a role in helping people to adapt to their limitations. The promotion of health, rather than dependence, is an important role for all health professionals.

Psychological ageing

An understanding of human psychology increased greatly during the twentieth century. Early theories of psychology, such as the work of Freud, were widely discussed (if sometimes misunderstood) by society as a whole, but the growth of psychology ironically contrasted with reduced public awareness of its development. Current theories of psychology are, in lay terms, relatively unfamiliar. Chapter 7, therefore, outlines the main, current theories of psychological ageing, with particular emphasis on the work of Erikson. This is developed to show how cognitive function, individuality and social relationships contribute to psychological health. Healthy psychological ageing is illustrated through such developments as the University of the Third Age.

Dementia is probably the most feared part of growing old. Yet the myths surrounding ageing, that it is synonymous with dementia, are nothing more than stereotypes. Increasingly, the importance of 'normal' or 'healthy' ageing has been emphasized. The stresses of life itself can contribute towards causing the development of dementia (Kitwood 1997). Therefore, healthcare has moved away from institutional care to seeking to support and maintain normal function and abilities. Health-care for older people is not just about the provision of hospital beds, but a range of multi-professional community and outpatient-hospital services that enable people to live as normal a life as possible.

However, while dementia should not be viewed as 'normal', it would be equally foolish to deny its existence. Chapter 8 therefore explores abnormal aspects of psychological ageing, with particular focus on:

- Alzheimer's disease
- Vascular dementia
- Dementia with Lewy bodies.

Physiology, psychology and sociology are interdependent; so contexts are given to show how factors from other sections of this book influence psychological health and can cause psychological ageing to become abnormal. For instance, assessing the problem is a necessary step to providing individualized healthcare; yet the assessment tools widely used within healthcare can be culturally biased, giving a falsely low impression of the cognitive abilities of people from ethnic minorities.

Sociological ageing

Sociological ageing affects the way in which people are viewed by others as they become older, the way in which they view themselves, and, there-fore, the way they interact with, and are treated by, society. Having explored issues around physical and psychological health in previous sections, the final section of this book provides a context for understand-ing social function and social health. Chapter 9 outlines the main theories of sociological ageing. For example, a simple, but significant, clue to the way older people are valued (or not) is betrayed not only by the language used with them but also by the attitudes of those around them. This includes the language and labels used about them. Words may begin as innocent descriptions of some phenomenon but, with repeated deroga-tory use, gain negative connotations. For example, 'elder' was once a term of veneration but now has negative connotations, and many people would prefer to be called 'old' or 'older'. Where possible, this wish has been respected throughout this book, the two exceptions being where replacing 'elder' would make the text grammatically clumsy or where the work of other authors is cited.

Arguably, ethics and morals should and do influence every human action. An increasing emphasis upon ethical (or unethical) actions within healthcare, together with an increasing emphasis on the individual accountability of each healthcare professional, has raised the profile of discussion about ethics within healthcare. Chapter 10 develops these issues, with particular focus on the ethical issues that surround ageing. Although ethical theory can initially appear rather abstract, its practical application can be illustrated by showing how healthcare can empower individuals with the ability to choose for themselves.

The UK, like most countries, is multi-racial. But, even within a single race, various cultures can exist. Therefore, if healthcare is to attempt to provide equal opportunities and access for all people within society, it must be culturally sensitive. However, the diversity of co-existing cultures can result in health professionals failing to meet the needs of some clients because they remain ignorant of their culture. It is important that staff working in a multi-cultural society such as the UK make positive efforts to extend their awareness of different cultural needs and know how those needs can be met in practice. The importance of this issue is raised in Chapter 11.

Other chapters of this book show ways in which health professionals can enhance the care provided to older people. But our actions are, at least in part, influenced by our own individual values and beliefs. Therefore, any study of healthcare will remain incomplete unless it explores the values and beliefs that motivate the people providing care. Everyone's individual values are partly influenced by the society and culture in which they develop, and by the people around them. Not surprisingly, the negative attitudes to ageing and older people that are identified in this book have resulted in largely negative attitudes among recruits to healthcare professions. This has contributed to the poor quality of care often given to older people. With an 'ageing population', this creates a challenge to both society and healthcare.

From the varying perspectives of this book, most of the chapters identify health problems that can occur with age. But health, rather than disease, should be, and often is, the norm. Chapter 13 therefore consolidates some of the key themes of this book: ageing should be healthy and healthcare should support people to live, and age, healthily rather than just treat the various diseases and problems that may occur.

So what can be done?

This book is primarily about, and for, healthcare practice. Some of the issues raised would need changes in society or at a governmental level. However, an awareness of these issues enables health professionals to provide better care. Therefore, the main emphasis in this book is on the actions that most health professionals can implement, whether through health promotion and education or through changing their own actions. Some of these changes, such as attitudes and language, cost little or nothing, although the difficulty of changing attitudes should not be underestimated.

Providing information to others through health promotion and education empowers other people to choose how they wish to live their lives. Ageing itself is irreversible, but changes in lifestyle may enable ageing to be healthy. Much discussion in this book has focused on older people, but ageing is something we are all experiencing all of the time. Knowing what factors may contribute to healthy and unhealthy ageing provides an opportunity to prevent problems before they (may) occur. Choices can range from major changes in lifestyle (such as increasing exercise to reduce the risk of heart disease) to relatively simple ones (such as taking calcium supplements to reduce the risk of osteoporosis). Health professionals have a duty to promote health and so may make this knowledge available through health-promotion initiatives. But information in books such as this may also be useful for the families and friends of older people. The authors of this book hope that readers will use the book not only to develop their knowledge for practice but also to develop their professional practice and to help themselves and others age healthily.

Conclusion

This book explores ageing from a range of physiological, psychological and sociological perspectives. Although ageing can be a negative experience, there has been frequent emphasis that ageing is a process and not a disease. It is possible, and desirable, to live healthily. Ageing is inevitable, but it is nothing to be ashamed about. We are all growing older. We can all hope that we shall grow old healthily. That hope is more likely to be achieved if we encourage healthy ageing, both for ourselves and for others. This fundamental aim is especially important for healthcare and health professionals. Themes covered in previous chapters of this book are summarized in this final chapter to emphasize the central issues raised.

Empathy, through 'gut feelings' of what we would like for ourselves or our own family and friends, can provide a useful guide for care. Kitwood (1995 p11) talks about the 'power to know, to discover, to give, to create, to love'. Empathy and gut feelings have a valid place in healthcare. But individual professional accountability also requires a sound knowledge base for practice and the need to examine the evidence base for care given (DOH 1999). This book supports discussion with current evidence. However, the 'swampy lowlands' of practice (Schon 1991) may not always provide sufficient time to rationalize care. In view of this, it is important for health professionals to take every opportunity to evaluate and re-evaluate the evidence for their own practice whenever possible. Practice is inevitably influenced by individual values and beliefs.

Individual health is a complex interaction between physical, psychological and social factors. Understanding these factors in depth, but also as a whole, can enable health professionals to encourage and promote healthy ageing. This text emphasizes the importance of the individual but also shows how social influences and beliefs affect healthcare provision and individual health. To this end, healthcare services should aim to provide the best possible conditions to help each *individual* to live and age healthily.

References

DOH (1999) Making a Difference. London: Department of Health.

Kitwood T (1995) Cultures of care: tradition and change. In: Benson S and Kitwood T The New Culture of Dementia Care pp. 7–11. London: Hawker Publications.

Kitwood T (1997) Dementia Reconsidered. Buckingham: Open University Press.

Schon D A (1991) The Reflective Practitioner. Aldershot: Arena.

Tinker A (1997) Older people in modern society 4th edn. London: Longman.

Glossary

acetylcholine (ACh) one of many chemicals used during transmission of signals in the nervous system; acetylcholine inhibits impulses and so is classified as an inhibitory neurotransmitter

adipose fatty tissue

affective (*psychology*) subjective feeling or emotional tone often accompanied by body expressions noticeable to others

agnosia failure to recognize or identify objects despite intact sensory function

alveolir the sacs in the lungs where exchange between gases in air breathed in and gases within the blood occurs.

anabolism building up of body tissue (usually used when discussing muscle mass)

androgens male hormones (e.g. testosterone)

angina a sharp stabbing chest pain caused by myocardial ischaemia

aphasia impairment or loss of ability to articulate words or comprehend speech

apoptosis programmed cell death (see Chapter 2)

apraxia impaired ability to carry out motor activities despite intact motor function

aqueous humour a type of watery fluid that fills the part of the eye in front of the lens (see 'vitreous humour')

arterioles small blood vessels between arteries and capillaries that control flow of blood into capillaries through dilating or constricting

aspiration pneumonia this is caused by stomach contents (which include hydrochloric acid that destroys cells lining the lungs) flowing or being regurgitated back up the oesophagus and entering the lower airways.

Healthy cough or gag reflexes would remove any stomach contents entering the airway; so people are at special risk to aspiration pneumonia if cough or gag reflexes are impaired (e.g. unconsciousness, CVA).

ATP (adenosine triphosphate) intracellular energy

atrial fibrillation cardiac dysrhythmia causing pulse to be irregular. Atrial fibrillation is the most common cardiac dysrhythmia and is frequently controlled with Digoxin.

atrioventricular node part of the cardiac conduction system

autocatalysis self-breakdown (i.e. self-destruction); this occurs when one chemical reaction triggers the next in a long sequence, resulting in destruction of the tissues/organ in which this occurs

calculus (plural = calculi) a stone formed within part of the body, for example renal calculi = kidney stones

carcinoma malignant tumour/cancer

cellular 'of cells', for example cellular apoptosis = apoptosis occurring within cells

cell line all succeeding generations of similar cells which derive from a cell type

cross-linking when structures that are normally separate join together. Increased cross-linking is seen with advancing age, but whether cross-linking is a cause or effect of ageing, and the extent to which external factors such as diet contribute to it, remains debatable.

cyanosis blue tinge to skin and mucous membranes caused by lack of oxygen in the blood. Cyanosis is best seen in nail beds and lips.

cytokines cell-killing components of the immune system. There are many different cytokines in the body, including interleukins.

diabetic retinopathy disease of the retina (at the back of the eye) resulting from diabetes mellitus. Diabetic retinopathy can cause severe visual impairment and blindness.

dysphasia difficulty speaking (usually, loss of the ability to speak). Dysphasia is most often caused by a stroke.

dysrhythmia an abnormal heart rhythm. (NB: many texts use 'arrhythmia' instead of 'dysrhythmia' but this is a grammatically incorrect label for any abnormal rhythm except for asystole)

embolus (plural = emboli) something circulating in the bloodstream that can obstruct small blood vessels. Emboli can be blood clots, air/gas or fat.

endocardium the inner lining of the heart; smooth simple squamous epithelium

erythrocytes red blood cells

free radicals any atom that has an unpaired electron or neutron in its outer orbit, for example oxygen molecules normally exist in pairs (O_2) but can exist as a radical (O) or superoxide (e.g. O_3). Radicals are very unstable and so only exist for microseconds before further chemical reactions. However, the sequence of chemical reactions is often many thousands of events long, resulting in significant damage to body tissues. Oxygen radicals, which pose the greatest threat to health, are normally controlled by antioxidant chemicals within the body, but with severe illnesses these antioxidant defences fail. Antioxidant supplements are available (e.g. from most chemists).

genitourinary the part of the urinary system shared with the reproductive (genital) system

glycosuria sugar in urine

homeostasis process of maintaining or restoring the body's normal internal environment

hypercalcaemia (hyper = high, calcaemia = blood calcium) high levels of blood calcium – normal blood calcium = 2.25–2.65 mmol/litre

hyperglycaemia high blood sugar (>8 mmol/litre)

hypertrophy enlargement

hypocalcaemia (hypo = low, calcaemia = blood calcium) low levels of blood calcium – normal blood calcium = 2.25–2.65 mmol/litre

hyponatraemia low levels of blood (plasma) sodium. Hyponatraemia is usually caused by excessive sodium loss, such as from vomiting, diarrhoea or excessive diuresis.

hypothalamus part of the brain stem; contains the vital centres controlling breathing, heart rate and the tone of blood vessels

hypoxia low levels of oxygen in the blood

insults in medical usage, an insult to a body system is damage caused to it

interleukin Cell-killing proteins that form part of the immune system (and are differentiated by number, e.g. interleukin 1, abbreviated as IL–1). Different interleukins have varied, but often powerful, effects of body function, many of which can aggravate diseases.

ischaemia lack of blood supply

kcal (kilocalorie) a unit of measurement for energy in foods

kyphosis excessive curving of the thoracic spine

Lewy bodies abnormal substances found in the mid-brain and brainstem of people with various organic brain diseases, such as Alzheimer's disease

macular degeneration degeneration of the maculae (part of the eye), which can be caused by various diseases, including diabetes mellitus

melanocytes cells that produce melanin

melanin a dark (black or brown) pigment responsible for hair, skin and pupil colouring. Age-related reduction in melanin production causes loss of hair colour in many older people, leaving hair grey or white

mitochondria part of the cell; mitochondria produce energy for the cell

mitosis production of cells by division

myocardial infarction death of heart muscle, i.e. heart attack

myocardium the middle layer of the heart, containing muscle

necrosis death of an area of tissue

neuroendocrine ('neuro' = nervous system, endocrine = hormone) effects on the nervous system, for example adrenaline stimulates the sympathetic nervous system, resulting in (among other effects) increased heart rate and blood pressure

nonstochastic something involving predetermination. Theories of ageing (see Chapter 2) are often classified as either 'stochastic' (random) or 'nonstochastic' (predetermined).

olfactory anything associated with the sense of smell

ototoxic (oto = ear) toxic to hearing

parathormone hormone produced by the parathyroid glands; parathormone increases blood calcium levels

pericardium outer layer of the heart; tough, fibrous tissue

peristalsis rhythmic muscle contraction causing movement of substances through (some) body systems

personhood (*psychology*) standing or status bestowed upon one person by another within a social context

reserve function the excess ability of a system to function over the minimum level of function needed to maintain homeostasis

sequela (plural = sequelae) consequence, usually used when describing adverse effects of diseases or treatments

shearing two forces (or pressures) working in opposition to each other

somaticize (*psychology*) to believe mistakenly that an emotional pain is a physical symptom

somatic mutation ('soma' = body) mutation of the body (i.e. mutation of body cells)

squamous scale-like, smooth layers of cells, such as those lining the cardiovascular system

stochastic random, as opposed to predetermined (see 'nonstochastic')

substantia nigra part of the brain. The inhibitory neurotransmitter dopamine is produced in the substantia nigra; failure of the substantia nigra to produce sufficient dopamine results in Parkinson's disease.

tumour necrosis factor alpha (TNFα) anti-cancer protein produced by the body in response to toxic substances, such as bacteria causing an infection. As well as protective effects, it can have serious, sometimes life-threatening, effects, including shock.

tunica adventitia outer layer of blood vessels; tough, fibrous tissue

tunica intima the inner layer of blood vessels, smooth thin simple squamous epithelium

tunica media the middle layer of blood vessels, containing muscle

vasomotor (the motor) part of the nervous system that controls vascular tone (e.g. vasoconstriction or vasodilation of arterioles). One of the two cardiac centres in the brainstem is the vasomotor centre, which, as its name implies, regulates this function.

venules small vessels between capillaries and veins, which regulate blood flow out of capillaries in a similar way to how arterioles regulate blood flow into capillaries

vestibulo-ocular and righting reflexes the main organs of balance are the semicircular canals in the inner ear (also called the 'vestibule'). The sense of balance is modified by other cerebral inputs, especially sight (ocular). Therefore, someone with healthy vestibule and ocular reflexes will usually manage to restore ('right') their body position to prevent falling.

vitreous humour a thick, jelly-like fluid that fills the eye behind the lens (see 'aqueous humour')

Index